MASTER THE KETTLEBELL

*How to Develop High-Level Skills in Movement,
Power Generation and Strength—
Using the World's Single Best Tool for the Job*

MAX SHANK, MASTER RKC

MASTER THE KETTLEBELL

How to Develop High-Level Skills in Movement, Power Generation and Strength—Using the World's Single Best Tool for the Job

A Dragon Door Publications, Inc. production
All rights under International and Pan-American Copyright conventions.
Published in the United States by: Dragon Door Publications, Inc.
5 East County Rd B, #3 • Little Canada, MN 55117
Tel: (651) 487-2180 • Fax: (651) 487-3954
Credit card orders: 1-800-899-5111 • Email: support@dragondoor.com • Website: www.dragondoor.com

ISBN 10: 0-938045-95-4   ISBN 13: 978-0-938045-95-3
This edition first published in December, 2014
Printed in China

Book design and cover by Derek Brigham • www.dbrigham.com • bigd@dbrigham.com
Photography by Don Pitlik

— CONTENTS —

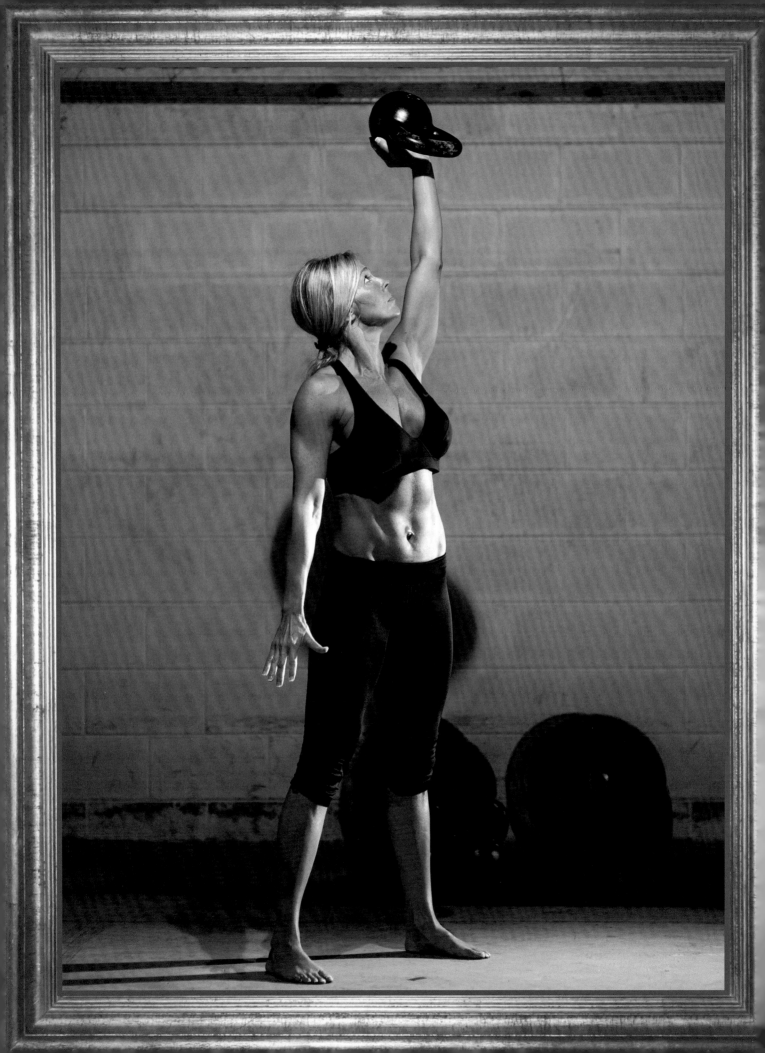

FOREWORD
by John Du Cane

YOUR BODY IS YOUR GOLD

Dragon Door was founded in 1991 to share my enthusiasm for Chinese internal martial arts, qigong and alternative healing systems in general. But growing up I had been a competitive athlete—breaking my school's long jump record and running like the wind in track. My two fellow track team buddies both achieved fame in their own way: Nick Drake became, posthumously, a massive musical cult figure. Mark Phillips became an Olympic gold-medal-winning horseman and married Princess Anne. All three of us, at the time, shared a common drive to excel physically and to WIN. The word "athlete", in fact, derives from the Greek verb "compete for a prize". We strove for the external gold of acclaim and recognition —and for the pride of achievement.

However, after being exposed to Yoga and various spiritual disciplines, my athletic vision morphed from "wanting to beat the other guys" to wanting to cultivate my athleticism simply for the glory of self-refinement. My own body became a prize in and of itself—a work of art to cultivate as an ongoing life-process. My body became the gold to process alchemically from baser stuff... My preferred disciplines in bodyweight exercise, Qigong and Tai Chi rewarded me with excellent posture, elegant movement and a balanced physique. I was ripped and reasonably muscular but nothing over the top. I wasn't competing, I was cultivating healthy strength and mobility as ends in themselves.

Lifting weights had always been an on-again, off-again complement to my main energetic and physical practices. It wasn't until Dragon Door originated the modern kettlebell movement in 2001, that I began to fall in love with weight lifting as a core method for enhancing healthy strength and healthy movement. The beauty of the kettlebell is that it dramatically enhances power generation through its emphasis on the explosive hip-drive and gives you a superb overall strength and conditioning challenge. I love that! The older I get, the more I value quality movement and the internally-oriented, health-focused exercise of the joints and tendons, as much as the muscles. The older I get, the more I now also revere the health-strength benefits of vigorous, skilled exercise with free weights. And NO free weight tool beats the kettlebell in bang-for-the-buck value, when to comes to radical physical transformation and the ongoing maintenance of that transformation. I mean, nothing comes close.

Fast forward to 2013 and Dragon Door's famed RKC kettlebell program took an historic leap forward in sophistication. With Dragon Door's more ambitious mission in place to have a major impact on global health, the RKC broadened and deepened its curriculum and placed a far greater emphasis on the importance of graduating instructors who were not only skilled athletes but skilled coaches. Dragon Door actively recruited and promoted men and women who role-modeled the impact of skillful kettlebell training, the RKC way. These men and women have lean, superb physiques and excellent movement skills. These men and women OWN the kettlebell as a tool for transforming the human body in every dimension. These men and women—the RKC leadership—possess deep coaching skills and a deep passion to ensure their clients achieve their desired transformational goals. Gone are the days of any self-centered, pseudo-militaristic bluster and punitive beat downs. The new, upgraded culture is tough but respectful—as a truly professional teaching culture should be. The approach is welcoming, helpful, good-natured and inclusive.

Now, no one in this resurgent RKC better exemplifies the new model of excellence than my good friend Max Shank. Max turned heads in dramatic fashion when he Tamed the Beast—and joined an elite fraternity capable of performing three very different lifts with a 48kg kettlebell: the press, the pistol and the pull up. For his preeminent skill in bodyweight exercise, Max was one of only two athletes selected to star in Paul Wade's **Convict Conditioning** video series, shot in Alcatraz. His evident teaching skills saw him rapidly promoted in the RKC leadership. As a Master RKC, Max has represented Dragon Door in Sweden, Italy, Germany and Australia, as well as the United States—and in every instance the praise for his teaching style has been off the charts. Lately, Max has been challenging for World Records in the Highland Games…

There are many reasons, then, that I am proud to introduce you to Max Shank, through his superb first book, *Master the Kettlebell.* You will see immediately from the photographs illustrating the book, that Max is indeed a magnificent athletic specimen—combining a great physique with impressive strength and terrific form. Study Max—either in this book or in person—and if you replicate what you see, athletic gold awaits you. As importantly, you'll be rewarded in *Master the Kettlebell* with an absolutely fluff-free blueprint on how to develop your own high-level skills in movement, power generation and strength—using the world's single best tool for the job.

I appreciate Max Shank for his supreme dedication to the art of HEALTHY, high-functioning, all-around athletic proficiency. And I welcome him proudly into the ranks of Dragon Door's already prestigious roster of authors!

Finally, let me express my gratitude to and admiration for the contribution made by Beth Andrews to *Master the Kettlebell*. In many ways, Beth Andrews is the perfect female complement to Max. Beth is only one of five women to achieve the women's version of the Beast Tamer Challenge, known as the Iron Maiden—same three lifts, but with a 24kg kettlebell. Like Max, Beth is the perfect role model physically for what can be achieved with the RKC kettlebell program. Currently a Senior RKC and a PCC Team Leader, Beth is an exemplary coach of the highest order. Other women the world over are inspired by her and strive to emulate her strength and form. Most men can only dream to match her athletically…☺ The photos of Beth in *Master the Kettlebell* say it all.

Thanks Beth! Thanks Max! As the saying goes: You're Golden…

In Health and Strength,

John Du Cane

John Du Cane

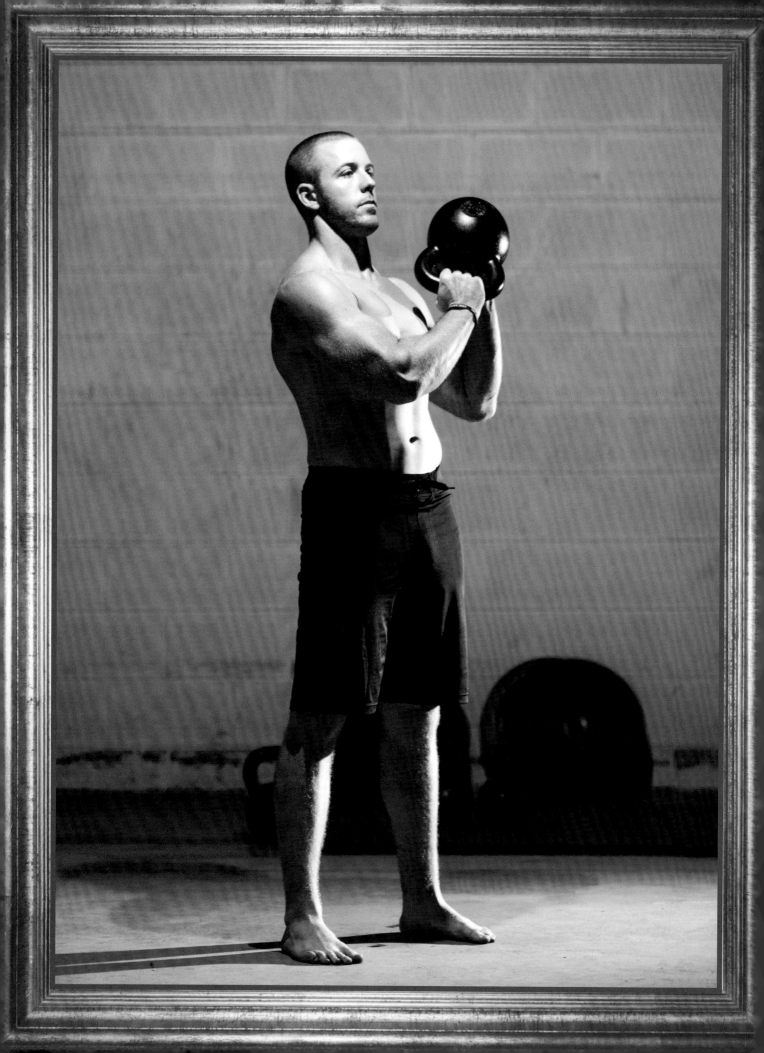

INTRODUCTION

WHY KETTLEBELLS?

Although kettlebell training has been around for hundreds of years, it's only recently become popular in the US. In an era of fitness machines that fail to deliver results, the American public has become sedentary, ill-nourished, and obese. Something must change before we regress even further. That change can be found in a return to basic physical fitness. Basic physical fitness can be described as the ability to move in a coordinated, unimpeded way while meeting the required demands of everyday life. Whether the situation is lifting a bag of groceries or getting up from the floor, the movements involved should be coordinated, unimpeded, and—most important—pain-free. The return to physical fitness can be achieved through kettlebell training.

Many of us are required to sit for extended periods of time because of our jobs and technology. I'm not going to tell someone to stop sitting at a desk job that supports their family, but the seated position is not ideal for our bodies. Lack of movement causes many problems that will be addressed later, but suffice it to say, most people are unable to move well and without pain.

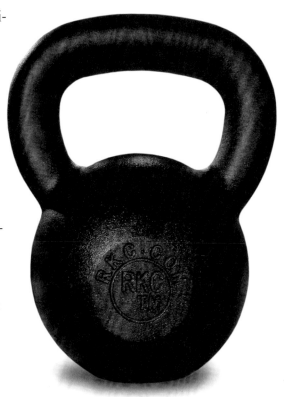

To make matters worse, exercise has been reduced to working out on a series of seated "torture devices". After sitting for 8 hours at a desk, we sit at the gym. After a half-hearted effort, we sit in the car to drive home where we once again perform the sacred act of sitting on our favorite couch.

We are bipedal—meant to walk and stand on two legs. Luckily, some of us have led the return to the past glory of true physical fitness with kettlebell training. Kettlebell training provides all the same benefits of regular free weights (dumbbells, barbells) plus a lot more. Kettlebells encourage and allow movement and stabilization in three dimensions. This results in a coordinated, synergistic body capable of performing any task without impediment or pain.

The magic of kettlebell training comes from its ability to create desirable movement patterns while efficiently enhancing physical capabilities and aesthetics. Most people would agree that exercise is a good thing, but exercise must be productive—every time you exercise, you must progress. Kettlebells are truly amazing because they are maximally efficient for fat loss or muscle gaining goals. Any athlete can use kettlebells to improve their overall athleticism—in any sport. Performed correctly, kettlebell training can change someone's life—as they learn to move well for the first time.

From this point on, you are not just a trainer, you are an instructor. You understand the most important concept in this entire book—why we train with kettlebells. You are not a zombie who only follows instructions and copies exercise programs for clients from a book. The most important thing to consider when considering true fitness, is to understand why you are performing a particular exercise—and what the result will be. As my friend Dan John says, "The goal is to keep the goal, the goal."

As a kettlebell instructor, you must understand why you are prescribing an exercise and what it will do. This book will give you many of the necessary tools to change a client's lifestyle, and the understanding of how and why these tools work. It will also teach you how and when to apply its concepts and will show you how to truly help people towards any of their goals.

WHY EXERCISE?

As of this writing, there are no magic pills for six pack abs, no super drinks for the strength to lift cars, and the only cure for an aching shoulder is usually a cortisone shot. But, with proper exercise (and nutrition), you can have incredible health, strength, and flexibility—while looking and feeling amazing! As a kettlebell instructor, your goal is to deliver these qualities with the methods in this book—and to understand why they work.

As with all forms of training, it is absolutely imperative to build on a good foundation. In the current personal training industry, there's often no assessment or preparation before "working out." At best this leads to mediocre results, and at worst, injury. When someone comes to you looking for results—no matter what their specific goal might be—you should be able to deliver. By performing a basic assessment of the client and implementing simple measures to insure their health and fitness, you are doing yourself and your client a great service.

Movement quality is an often overlooked or completely ignored aspect of the current fitness paradigm. Kettlebells do an excellent job of helping people re-learn ideal movement dynamics. Ideal movement is the ability to squat, lunge, or reach your arms over your head without straining. It means that you can move smoothly and effortlessly through a wide range of motion. Kettlebells help people move better.

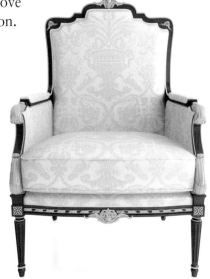

One major source of movement dysfunction is *the chair*. Chairs put people in a hip-flexed, glute-relaxed position for hours at a time. This effectively shortens the hip flexors and encourages gluteal amnesia—leading to some of the postural/movement dysfunctions that can become serious problems when ignored. The following chapter will address assessment, corrections of common dysfunctions, and a dynamic warm up that—when combined with proper kettlebell training—will yield amazing results for you and your clients.

FROM THE GROUND UP—LINKAGE AND INTERMUSCULAR COORDINATION

Building a complete athlete (or human being) really starts from the ground up. We are dependent on our ability to coordinate and align many moving parts. Beginning with the feet and moving upward, it is important for the joints to be mobile and stable. The movement of our joints cannot be inhibited, and they must support the body parts above and below it. The mobility section of this book will give us the movement and range of motion critical to moving the way we are built to move.

Acquiring intermuscular coordination is the next task in building an exceptionally functioning human body. Intermuscular coordination is the ability to synchronize multiple muscle groups to perform large, compound movements like jumping, squatting, or pulling.

Many training programs are built around isolating then growing or strengthening individual muscles. This mode of training will accomplish that goal, because the body adapts to all training. But, by neglecting compound movements that incorporate multiple joints and muscles, the trainee ends up with a "Frankenstein" body—a collection of parts that are individually strong, but without coordination or the ability to work together. An all-star team is a similar example, the team may have all the best players (statistically speaking), but they aren't effective as a team because they don't know how to play well together. Our methods will emphasize intermuscular coordination, and full body movements.

BONES, MUSCLES, JOINTS, TENDONS, LIGAMENTS

Smart strength training also improves the durability and strength of your soft and hard tissues. Wolff's Law states that a bone will re-model (strengthen) across lines of stress. It also shows that a healthy bone, when put under no stress, will weaken significantly. Davis' Law essentially states the same for soft tissues including muscles, tendons, and ligaments. Weight training—especially with kettlebells—is an essential element for promoting orthopedic longevity.

Wolff's and Davis' Laws go hand in hand with the SAID principle, Specific Adaptation to Imposed Demands. This principle simply states that the body, via the nervous system, will adapt to become more efficient (better) at whatever it practices with the highest frequency and intensity.

Sitting down for 12 hours a day? Your body will adapt to sitting. Doing tons of crunches? Your body will adapt to that position. Remember when Mom said your face would "freeze like that" if you kept making faces? She was sort of right—you would just have to do it a lot longer to see the change!

As you train, these laws are always in effect. Your body will adapt to what you do with it, and to the positions you're in. These combined ideas are the foundation for success in physical strength and wellness. Awareness of them should change your approach to training yourself and others.

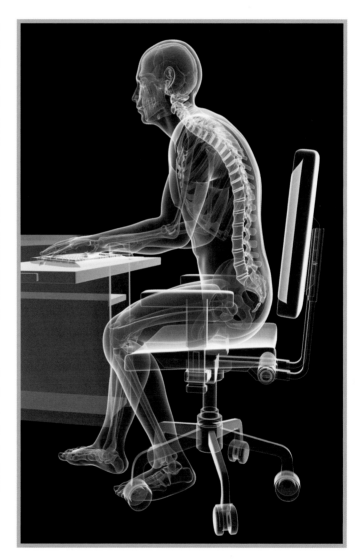

CHAPTER ONE

FIRST TIME CLIENT ASSESSMENT

The following should only be done after obtaining the client's full health history, and if necessary, a medical professional's permission to exercise.

NECK CLEARANCE:

While standing with feet together, have your client slowly perform the following neck movements:

- Flex
- Extend
- Rotate side to side
- Rotate and Flex both sides
- Tilt side to side

Remember to look for asymmetry (any discrepancies between the right and left sides). Any pain should be noted and referred to a medical professional unless it is resolved with thoracic and shoulder corrections elsewhere.

SHOULDER MOBILITY:

Have the client make thumbless fists before trying to touch their fists together by reaching one arm above their head, and the other arm behind their back in one motion. Don't allow them to crawl their fists together. Measure the distance between their fists on each side. The distance between fists should be within one and a half hand lengths (measure their hand). Look for asymmetry.

IMPINGEMENT TEST:

The client puts his or her hand on the opposite shoulder and lifts the elbow without removing the palm from the shoulder. If there is pain, the client should be referred to a medical professional.

THORACIC ROTATION:

The client takes a seated position (in a chair or cross-legged on floor if appropriate). With a dowel or PVC pipe touching both clavicles and while squeezing an object (a yoga block, phone book, rolled up towel, etc) between their knees to inhibit lumbar rotation, the client will rotate to one side as far as possible while maintaining good posture. Repeat on other side. Thoracic tightness can result in low back compensation and poor shoulder mobility. Note asymmetry if present.

TOE TOUCH:

Client stands with feet together and attempts to touch their toes without bending their knees.

SQUAT:

Client takes a stance with feet shoulder width apart and squats down until the crease of the hip is below the knee. Heels should stay on the ground and the toes, knees and hips should be in alignment. Look for knees caving inward, feet tilting in medial or lateral directions, heels leaving the floor, or the inability to drop hips below knees with good posture. The squat is scored as pass/fail.

LUNGE:

Client will assume a split stance on a line and descend into a lunge while keeping the front heel down and maintaining good (tall) posture. Repeat for both sides. Note any asymmetry.

GLUTE BRIDGE (SINGLE AND DOUBLE LEG):

The client will lay down on his or her back with both feet flat on the floor. Ask client to bridge as high as possible while pushing through their heels. The client's body should be a straight line from the knee to the shoulder, and in the hip flexor area.

Repeat with one leg pulled in to chest, then switch sides. Note any difference between double and single leg bridges, and left and right sides.

ANKLE DORSIFLEXION:

Place one foot 4 inches away from the wall. Then, while keeping the heel down, attempt to touch the front knee to the wall. If this is easily achieved, move back an inch at a time until the limit is reached. Repeat on other side and notice any asymmetry. If the client can't touch their knee to the wall when it is 4 inches away, this is an indication of a tight calf or lack of mobility in the joint itself—both can be improved by using this test as a mobility drill before exercise.

TRUNK STABILITY/UPPER BODY STRENGTH:

The client assumes a prone position on the floor and brings the heels of both hands in line with the chin (ladies' hands will be in line with the shoulder). Instruct the client to lift their knees and elbows off the floor while leaving their torso in contact with floor. Next, tell the client to move their body as one unit while performing a push-up. Watch for any swaying or "snaking" of the body, especially in the lumbar spine. If the client is unable to perform a solid push up as one unit, then they have poor stability through the anterior core.

Any of the tests performed in the initial assessment should be revisited often to measure progress and the effectiveness of the fitness program.

Now that we have a good idea of our client's physical abilities and restrictions, we can begin to build them up.

WHAT IS A TRIGGER POINT?

"A trigger point is a section of muscle that is unusually sensitive to pressure, resulting in a pinching or burning sensation when the area is compressed. This increases tension throughout the entire muscle and also can cause pain in another area of the body."
—Cook, *Athletic Body in Balance*

"A trigger point is a small area of muscle in a state of constant contraction that causes dysfunction within that muscle, with the possibility of 'triggering' other muscles (causing dysfunction in those muscles). Dealing with trigger points doesn't have to be complicated and is usually a simple endeavor. It will also give you instant credibility with your clients, because of its ability to get them moving better and out of pain quickly."
—Travell & Simmons, *The Trigger Point Therapy Manual*

RECOMMENDED TOOLS:

- Massage Stick
- Racquetball/Lacrosse Ball
- Golf Ball
- Foam Roller
- Thera Cane

Disclaimer: This book is not intended to be a comprehensive trigger point therapy manual. For more information regarding the subject, both *The Trigger Point Therapy Manual* by Travell/Simmons, or the more concise overview, *The Trigger Point Therapy Workbook* by Davies are strongly recommended. That said, the following is a plan for dealing with trigger points.

PREVENTION IS BETTER THAN REHABILITATION!

Starting from the feet upward, this is the protocol for releasing fascial adhesions:

The client begins by rolling out the bottom of their feet with a golf or tennis ball while holding onto something stable for balance. They should look for "hot spots" or trigger points and attempt to release the associated pain. Adhesions in the feet can cause dysfunction further up the kinetic chain. Because we are bipedal, the feet have a very high concentration of mechanoreceptors and are put under a lot of stress. Any trigger points or adhesions in the feet can be extremely detrimental to safety as well as performance. Rolling out the feet can be done frequently (i.e. under a desk at work) and can be beneficial in treating plantar fasciitis. Wearing high heels or other problematic shoes can exacerbate foot problems and make the feet especially tender. In some cases, it's recommended to start with a softer implement like a racquetball or tennis ball.

Using the massage stick (or PVC pipe), the client will start with their calves and work up the leg hitting the IT band, TFL, and quadriceps. They should use light strokes to probe for tender spots, as before.

For the larger areas like glutes, thoracic spine, hamstrings, a foam roller is preferred.

Clients are most likely to injure or lose mobility in their shoulders. Being sedentary (active for less than 8 hours per day—which describes almost everyone) creates trigger points in muscles from lack of use, especially related to shoulder flexion (arms overhead).

Shoulder mobility—in all its forms—is the bane of many fitness professionals. Too often, trainers will modify a program to avoid the shoulders instead of addressing and fixing the problem. Recognize that we are not physical therapists and cannot diagnose shoulder dysfunction. But, with practice, we can sometimes solve simple problems like trigger points in the traps and muscles of the rotator cuff—supraspinatus, infraspinatus, teres minor, subscapularis—the major culprits behind most shoulder pain and dysfunction.

Using the racquetball, lacrosse ball, or Thera Cane, probe the back of thc shoulder around the blade and the trapezius (upper and lower) looking for trigger points. Elimination of trigger points in the shoulder should be performed with the previously discussed techniques.

Using this sequence from head to toe as a precursor to exercise can help to avoid many problems and potential injuries.

KNOW THE RULES:

Make sure to understand the rules and laws regarding personal trainers touching or performing any kind of massage or manual therapy on clients. In some states it is illegal for personal trainers to touch clients with the intent of manual therapy. It is a good idea to make use of the available tools and teach your clients to do it themselves.

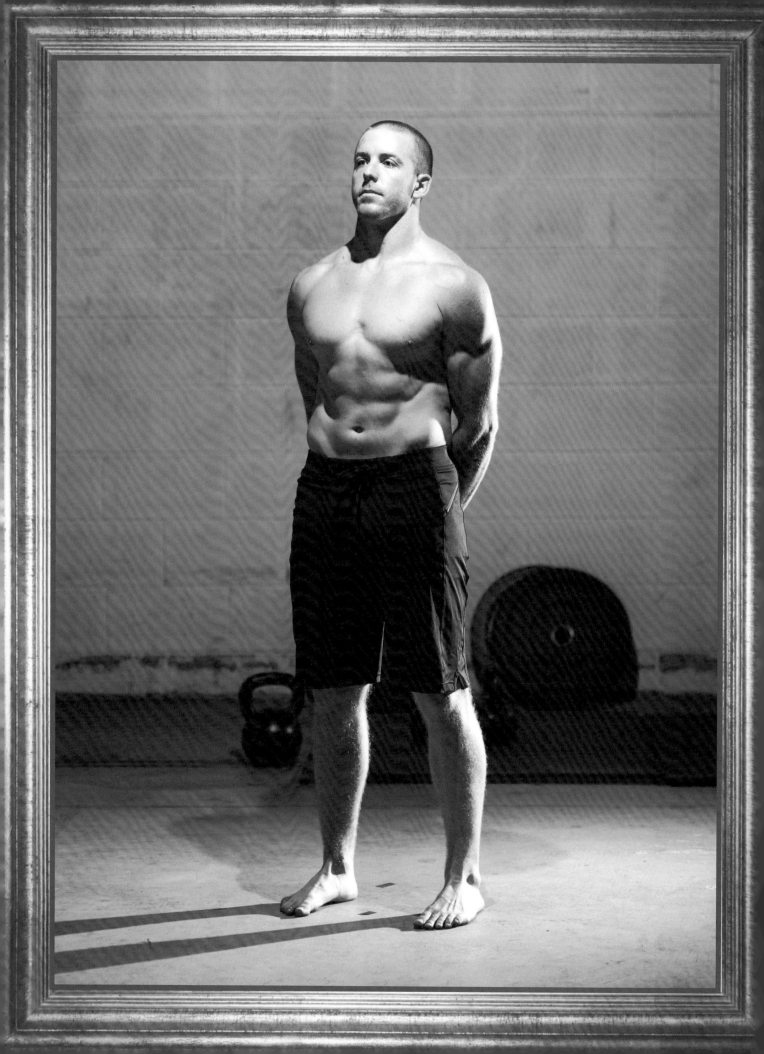

CHAPTER TWO

DYNAMIC WARM UP

Most warm ups include 5 minutes on the treadmill and a few half-hearted quad stretches. While it is important to increase core temperature and blood flow to initiate exercise, it's only part of the equation in warming up. Swings and get-ups (see Exercises section) and a simple head to toe joint mobility routine will cover all the bases in a warm up. It will also release tightness accumulated outside the gym, or reveal tightness you (or your client) weren't aware of that day.

THE BENEFITS OF A PROPER WARM UP INCLUDE:
- Increased speed of muscle contraction
- Increased muscle electrical activity
- Increased limit (maximal) strength
- Increased duration of muscular contractions
- Improvement in connective tissue's ability to accept force
- Reduction of potential injuries (Hatfield, *Fitness: The Complete Guide*)

Assume a tall standing position. Start with the neck mobility drills and move downward to the toes.

NECK
Up/Down
Rotate Side/Side
Tilt Side/Side

SHOULDERS
Circle (arms relaxed)
Circles (arms straight, forward and backward)

SPINE
Flex/Extend

HIPS
Hula Circles
Leg Swings

ANKLE
Dorsiflexion/Plantarflexion
Circles (Both Directions)

When the body is sufficiently warm and the joints are prepped for more vigorous activity, you may proceed into the day's training. However, it is recommended that a few more movements precede your "workout."

THE TURKISH GET-UP + ARM BAR + WINDMILL
This sequence of exercises is incredible for preparing a client for a serious lifting session. This sequence, plus some kettlebell swings to raise core temperature will prepare your client for any activity you can throw at them. But, it should only be used as a warm up if the client is already comfortable with the movements. See the Exercise section for a full description of each movement.

MOBILITY DRILLS TO PRECEDE ACTIVITY AND CORRECTIONS FOR INITIAL ASSESSMENT
Why bother identifying imbalances and weakness if you aren't going to try to fix them?! Here we will discuss how you are going to address those problems.

SIDE LYING THORACIC ROTATION

Lie on the floor on your side with a towel or pillow to support the head and neck. Place the top leg on a block or medicine ball so that the knee and hip are flexed to more than 90 degrees. From this position, rotate the upper body so that the top shoulder touches the floor behind you.

This is a terrific drill for opening up the thoracic spine, which can cause not only shoulder inflexibility, but overcompensation from the lumbar spine.

ACTIVE HAMSTRING STRETCH

Substantial research indicates stretching a muscle before activity will actually decrease its potential power output. But, if someone has hamstrings so tight that their mobility is inhibited, it's important to stretch before activity. We will use a PNF (Proprioceptive Neuromuscular Facilitation) contract-relax supine floor stretch. The trainer will assume a kneeling or half kneeling position with a hand or shoulder under the client's calf. First, the client will push away from the stretch while the trainer resists. Then while the client relaxes, the trainer will increase the stretch by a small amount. Repeat the process for the desired number of repetitions.

GOBLET SQUAT STRETCH

Often, a simple squat stretch can go a long way towards fixing a squat. Take a kettlebell by the horns (the sides of the handle) at chest level. Then, using the bell as counterweight, descend into a squat where the points of the elbows push against the vastus medialis. Hold the stretch for 5-10 seconds while spreading your elbows apart, then return to the start position by either setting the kettlebell down on the floor, or standing up as in a traditional squat (if appropriate for the client's fitness level).

HIP FLEXOR STRETCH AND GLUTE BRIDGES

Many problems in the lower body can be attributed to tight hip flexors and weak glutes. After all, we sit on our glutes all day with our hips in flexion. There are two recommended stretches for the hip flexors. First, the Thomas Test Stretch—also a test for hip flexor tightness. The client assumes a supine position at the edge of a massage table with their sacrum near the edge of the table. With a neutral sacrum, both hips flexed, and knees hugged into chest, the client will release and relax one leg. If it does not fall so that the femur and calf are parallel to the floor, then the hip flexor or quad are tight, respectively. From this position, stretch the lower leg in the direction of the ideal position.

The second stretch is a kneeling hip flexor stretch. Assume a half-kneeling position with the femur of the down leg perpendicular to the floor. The leg that's up should have the femur parallel to the floor, making a 90 Degree angle. From this position, contract the glutes and ease the hips forward while maintaining a tall posture. To increase the intensity of the stretch, put the back foot on a box or up against a wall.

After the hip flexor/quad stretch, perform a set of single leg bridges so the client owns the new range of motion and reassesses the relationship between the hip flexor ROM and glute strength. This sequence will often fix a poor lunge or squat from the initial screen.

SHOULDER STRETCH—PARTNER ARMBAR

(See the Exercise section for a description of the Kettlebell Armbar) The client will lay on the floor in a supine position with one arm raised in front of them and the other above their head on the floor. The client will grasp your hand. Instruct the client to roll over so that their hips face the floor and their head rests on their other arm. Remind the client to keep their shoulder from popping up toward their ear while you gently apply traction to the shoulder. It's normal to also experience a stretch in the thoracic spine, pectorals, and anterior deltoid during this mobility drill.

WALL SLIDE

The client will stand with their back and heels touching a wall. Instruct the client to push their elbows and wrists into the wall during shoulder flexion and elbow extension. It will look like the client is doing a press. The challenge is keeping the arms and wrists in contact with the wall during the exercise. This move will stretch the pectorals and engage the postural muscles on the back of the shoulders, including the rotator cuff and lower trapezius.

CONCLUSION

It is important to recognize the value of proper physical assessment and preparatory routine on a client's well being. It is also crucial to understand how to help clients achieve their goals safely and effectively.

CHAPTER THREE

THE
EXERCISES

When it comes to training with kettlebells, two exercises lay the foundation for everything else—the swing and the get-up. Smart implementation of the swing and get-up will build a rock solid foundation of physical capability from the shoulders down to the toes.

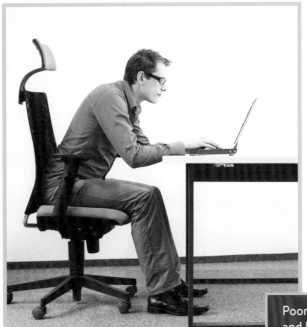

Poor posture: Hips flexed, kyphotic, and head jutted forward.

Understanding why the swing is so special requires an understanding of how people are supposed to move—and how they usually move. Modern man is sedentary relative to his evolutionary status. The human body is designed to be in motion—crawling, climbing, foraging, hunting, for the majority of our waking hours. Unfortunately, societal obligations often necessitate a sedentary lifestyle. Many jobs require sitting in front of a computer and being mentally productive while neglecting the physical body. Sitting down for long durations causes poor posture.

As you can see from the picture, sitting is not an ideal position. Coincidentally, this is also the same position that we're in while driving, eating, and watching TV. Hypothetically, someone might wake up, sit down to eat breakfast, sit down in the car on the way to work, sit down for 8 hours at work, sit down in the car on the way home, and finally sit down to eat dinner and watch TV for a few hours before finally going to sleep. When the body is subjected to a seated position for long periods of time, it begins to recognize that position as correct, and strives to maintain it instead of the ideal posture. The main effects of sitting are recognized in the tightening and shortening of the hip flexors, pectorals and shoulders, along with the sensory motor amnesia of the glutes, hamstrings, and back. Fortunately, the swing addresses all of the major problems caused by sitting and—for all intents and purposes—the swing is the exact opposite of sitting down in a chair.

During a properly performed kettlebell swing, the entire musculature of the backside is strengthened. Simultaneously, the muscles on the front half of the body—primarily the hip flexors and pectorals—are stretched. While sitting is a static hip flexed position, the swing is a dynamic hip extension. A process called reciprocal inhibition causes the simultaneous stretching of the antagonist muscles. Reciprocal inhibition occurs when an agonist (in this case, the glutes and hamstrings) contracts and causes its antagonist (the hip flexors) to relax, or to stretch. According to Gray Cook in *Movement*, reciprocal inhibition is the most efficient and effective way to initiate change in a dysfunctional pattern (266). Armed with this knowledge we can easily use the kettlebell to initiate a positive change in our clients' posture and movement quality.

First, have the client remove their footwear. The bottoms of our feet are loaded with mechanoreceptors that give feedback to your brain about your physical position in time and space. Wearing big shoes with a lot of padding is somewhat like trying to read Braille while wearing mittens. Also, shoes with cushions in the heel and forefoot create an unstable surface. When training with kettlebells, you want to be firmly rooted through the ground to improve safety as well as performance.

TEACHING THE SWING:

The bottom and top positions of a correctly performed kettlebell swing are identical to a proper RDL (Romanian Deadlift).

It's very important to allow your client to adapt to new positions when teaching them a brand new movement for the first time. Spending time in both the bottom and top positions of the deadlift—or any exercise you're teaching—will increase kinesthetic awareness. With some manual correction to these positions, most clients will be ready to proceed with the swing.

In spite of excellent instruction, some clients will have trouble feeling the correct positions for themselves. This being the case, it is your job to help with the following concepts and drills.

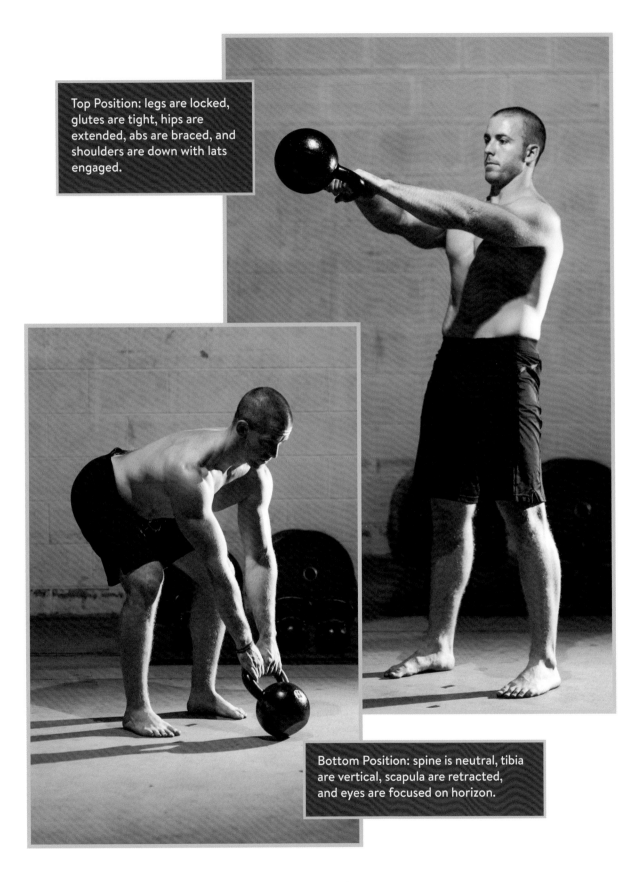

Top Position: legs are locked, glutes are tight, hips are extended, abs are braced, and shoulders are down with lats engaged.

Bottom Position: spine is neutral, tibia are vertical, scapula are retracted, and eyes are focused on horizon.

The bottom position of the deadlift is more challenging to correct. Many trainees will simply bend over to pick up the kettlebell. It is important to focus on learning a good hip hinge. A hip hinge happens when you fold at the torso and reach your hips behind you—in this drill, toward a wall.

The first technique to reinforce this is the Wall Swing Drill with Stick.

Instruct your client to hold the stick (PVC pipe or dowel—unweighted) so it touches the sacrum, thoracic spine, and head. If no equipment is available, an acceptable alternative is have them interlace their fingers behind their head with shoulders abducted. If that's not possible due to shoulder pain or other factors, have the client place their hands on their hips. Have the client stand 12-18 inches away from the wall and instruct them to reach back with their hips to touch the wall very lightly with their glutes. If the

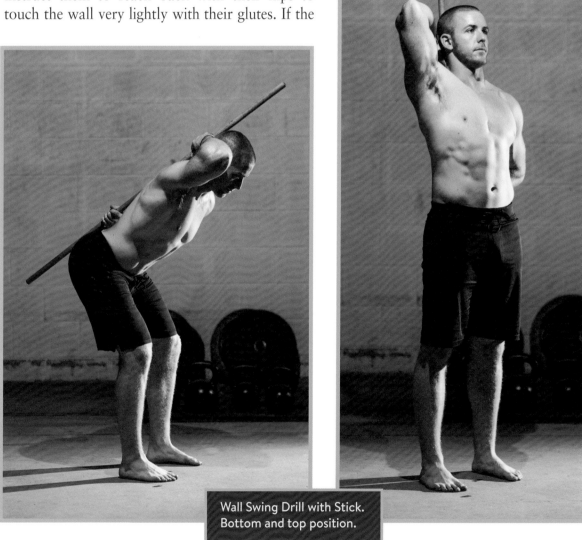

Wall Swing Drill with Stick.
Bottom and top position.

client leans up against the wall, they are not performing the drill correctly. While reaching back with their hips, the client should maintain a tall posture, and vertical shins. If the client flexes excessively at the knees (as in a squat) they will not reach the wall.

While instructing, convey an image of a bow and arrow for the hip hinge. Have the client imagine their hips are the bowstring which they must pull back to achieve maximum potential energy. Once a good top and bottom position have been achieved, instruct the client to make the movement more explosive by snapping their hips forward to the top position while simultaneously locking their knees. Once they are proficient, perform the same movement with a kettlebell. Use your judgment when choosing an appropriate weight, they should not have to struggle. 16kg for healthy men and 12kg for healthy women is usually appropriate.

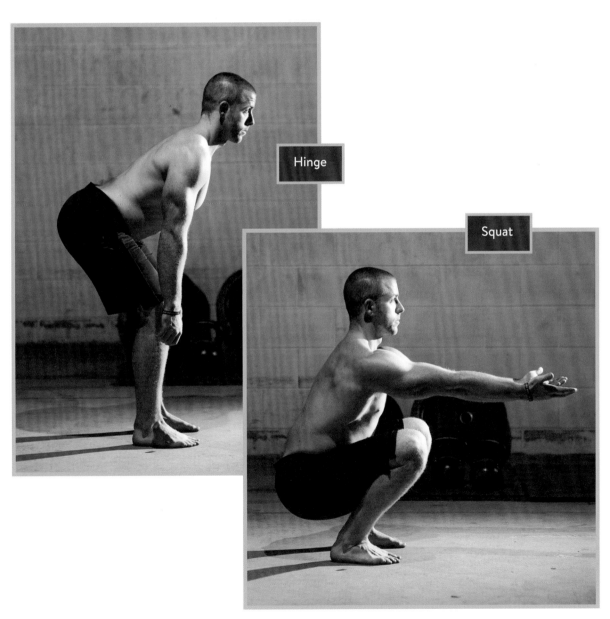

Hinge

Squat

Once the explosive deadlift has been achieved, you have the client perform the same movement with the kettlebell starting 6 inches behind them in the bottom position (credit goes to Zar Horton for this teaching method). When the client explodes to the top position, the bell will seem to float forward—which is the sensation that you want them to experience. Be sure to demonstrate enough swings so that they understand how the ideal form should look. Next, have the client perform a few repetitions starting with the kettlebell 6 inches behind their feet at the bottom position, explosively snapping the hips to the top position, then returning to the start position with the kettlebell. Once the client tries it without setting the bell down on the ground, they have done their first swing.

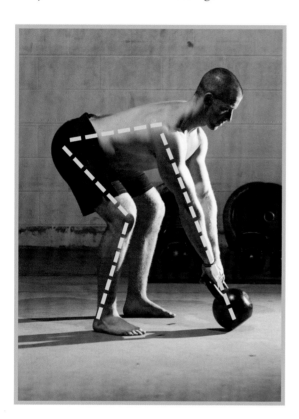

Once your client has reached this level of competence, you will want to refine their technique. Explain that hip flexion (folding back or hinging at the hips) should match the movement of reaching back with the kettlebell in the same area. The hip hinge shouldn't happen during the downward phase—until the upper arms contact the torso. Show the client to "throw the bell through the stomach and get out of the way."

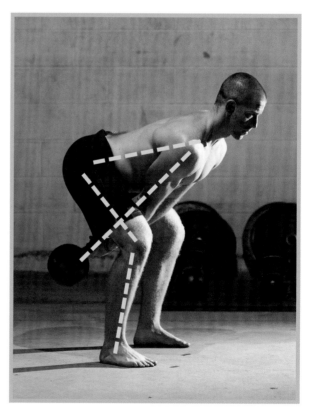

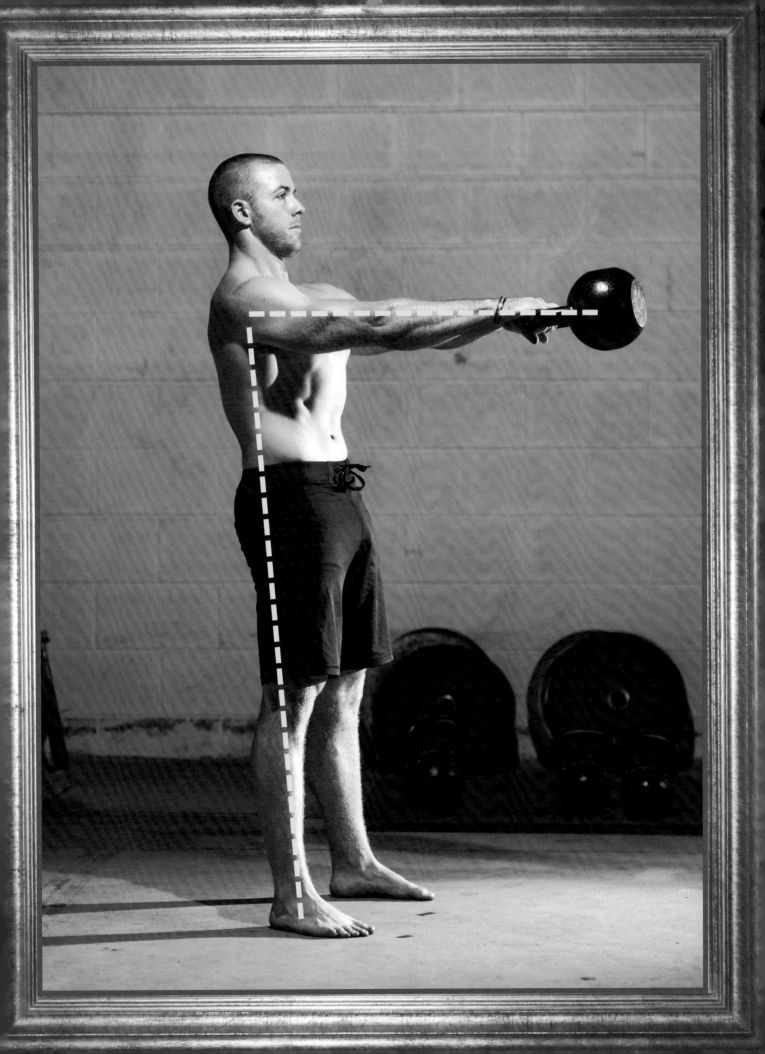

CHARACTERISTICS OF A GOOD KETTLEBELL SWING:

- No shoes (flat bottom shoes are acceptable but not ideal)
- Spine remains neutral or slightly extended throughout
- The movement of the kettlebell matches the movement of the hips
- Shins remain perpendicular to the floor
- There's always a straight line from the shoulder to the bottom of the kettlebell
- There's a vertical line from the head to the toe at the top position
- The glutes, abs, quads, and lats are engaged at the top position
- Heels and toes stay on the floor throughout the entire movement
- Scapulae are retracted throughout the movement

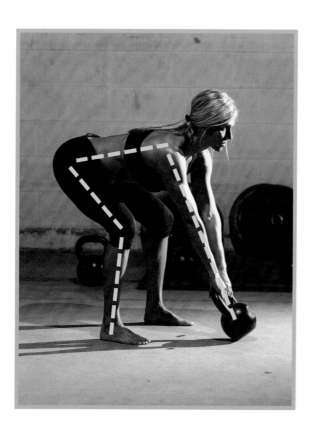

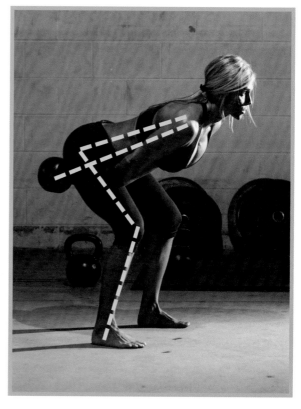

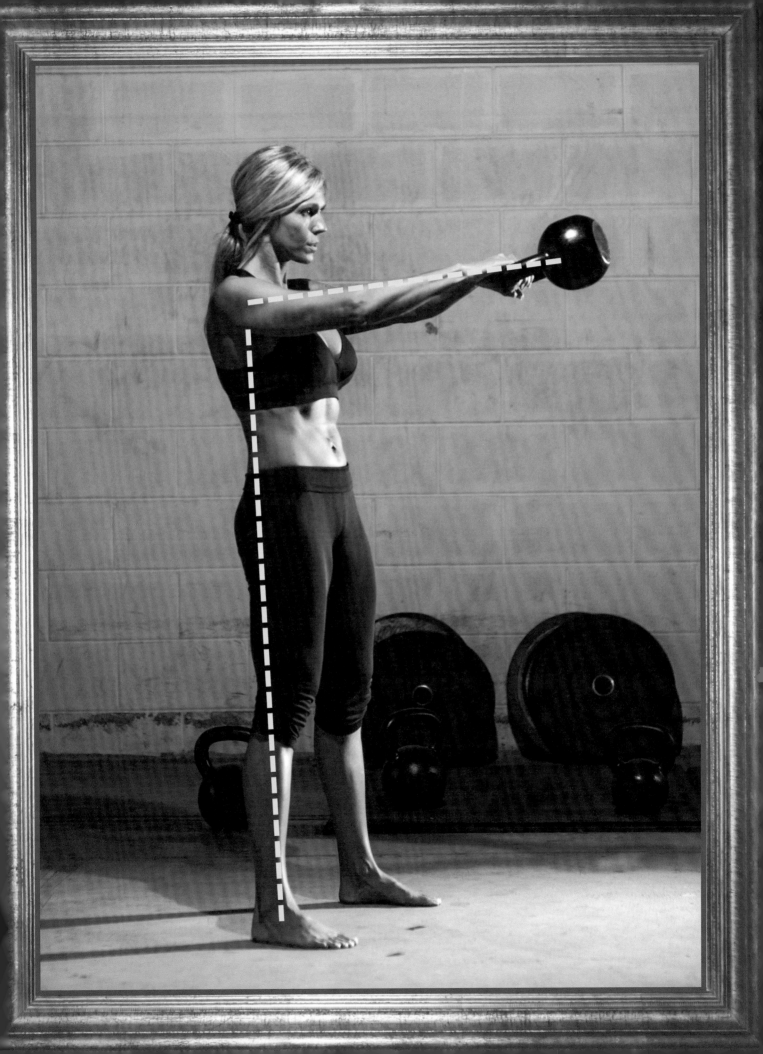

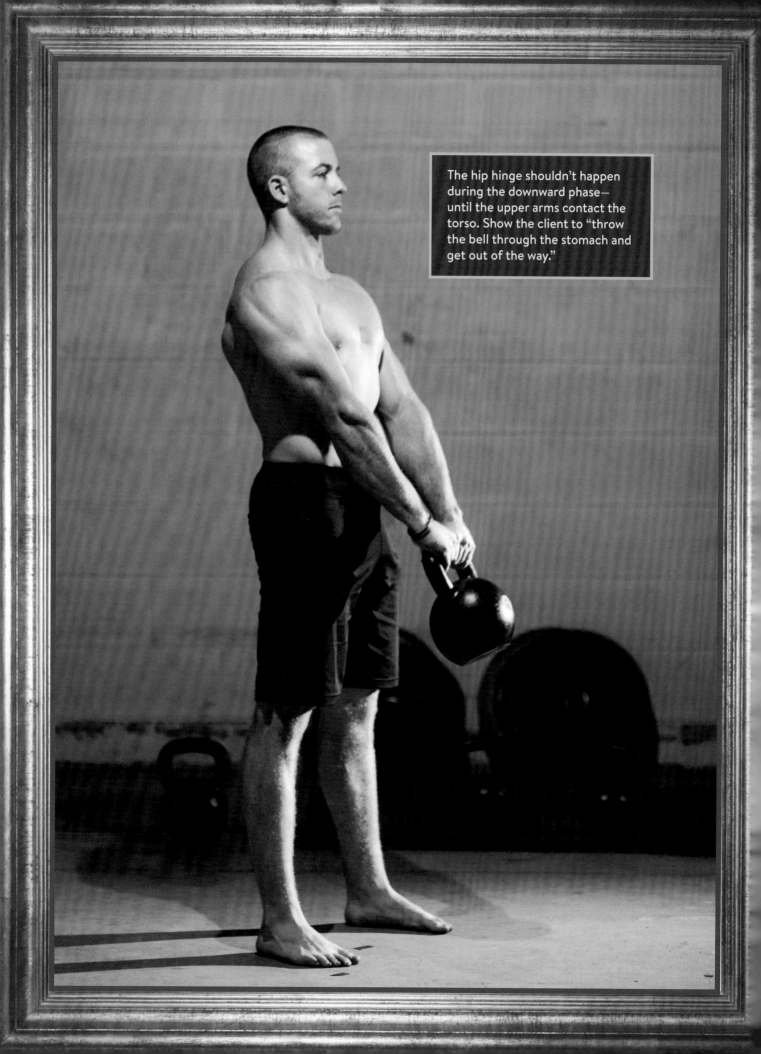

The hip hinge shouldn't happen during the downward phase— until the upper arms contact the torso. Show the client to "throw the bell through the stomach and get out of the way."

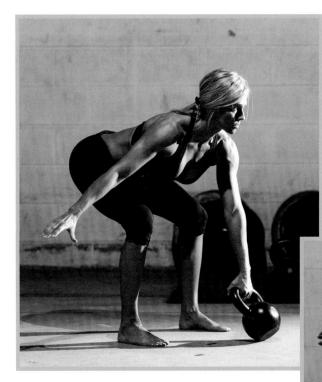

Some clients will run into problems during the swing. These mistakes should be corrected on an individual basis using specific drills to reinforce proper technique.

COMMON MISTAKE #1:

Lifting the kettlebell with the arms rather than the hips.

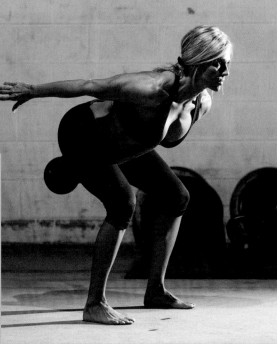

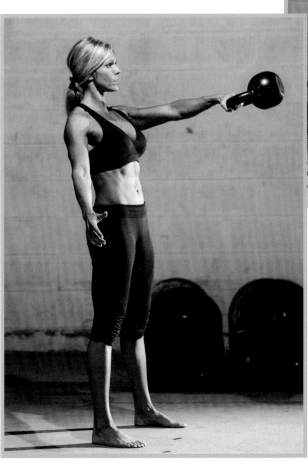

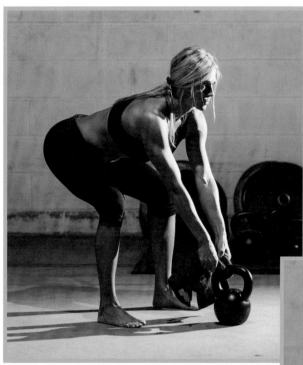

SOLUTION:

Towel Swing. Loop a towel around the kettlebell handle and grasp the ends of the towel close to the handle. Perform swings while maintaining a straight line from the shoulder to the end of the bell at all times.

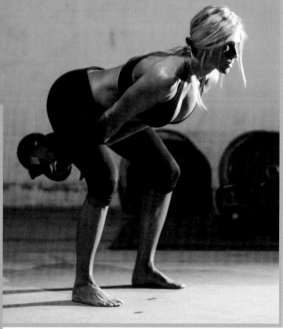

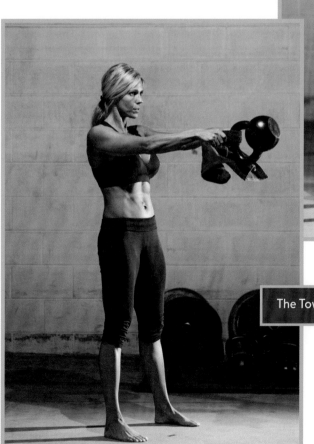

The Towel Swing.

COMMON MISTAKE #2:

The client squats instead of hinging at the hip during the backswing.

SOLUTION:

Explain to your client what you will be doing before trying this drill. Gently guide the kettlebell back between the legs during the downswing by giving it a little backwards push. Be sure the client keeps their shins parallel to the floor.

COMMON MISTAKE #3:

Sloppy lockout—including excessive backward lean and/or soft hips at extension.

SOLUTION:

Provide tactile feedback. Use discretion and explain the drill to your client first. At the lockout, lightly tap the client's belly and glutes with a fist to be sure they are forcefully contracted at the top of the swing. Explain to your client that without the forceful contraction, the lower back can be in a disadvantaged position with the potential for injury. If the client still struggles with the idea, they should practice a standard plank to help understand the feeling at the correct top position in an unloaded environment.

After the client has shown safety and competence in the two arm swing, you may teach them the one arm swing. All of the same rules apply as in the two arm swing, but only one hand is used to hold onto the bell. A common mistake with the one arm swing occurs when the working arm pulls forward during the swing. Instruct your client to quickly tap the handle of the kettlebell with their free hand at the top of the swing to easily fix this issue.

The swing is a terrific movement with many potential benefits. It's also the cornerstone of kettlebell training. At first, the movement will seem very awkward and unnatural for most people. It's important to be patient with your clients and spend plenty of time making sure that the proper movement is learned. When teaching the swing, keep the reps at 15 or less and give plenty of breaks in between sets. There's a greater chance of injury if these precautions are not observed.

THE GET-UP

The get-up is the second foundational kettlebell exercise. When combined with the kettlebell swing, it has the potential to build a strong, symmetrical, and injury-proof physique. The get-up increases movement quality and proprioception for the hips and shoulders while stabilizing the core.

At first glance, the get-up is sometimes dismissed as simply "standing up with a weight overhead." This is true, but misses the big picture. To properly teach and perform the get-up, it must be broken up into individual steps. This method insures a standard of safety, movement quality, and optimum performance.

STEP 1: ROLL TO PRESS

On the ground, instruct the client to roll to their right side, grab the kettlebell and bring it to their chest with both hands. From this position, the client will press the kettlebell to a full lock out. The scapulae should be retracted, depressed, and flat on the floor. A cue for this position is to think of pulling the scapulae into the opposite back pocket. The concept of "packing the shoulder" is required for proper overhead movement. If the rotator cuff, latissimus dorsi, and serratus do not actively pull the humerus downward during shoulder flexion, there's a risk of impingement at the acromioclavicular joint. The idea of shoulder packing should be made very clear in the first step, and maintained through every step and transition of the get-up as well as all overhead lifting.

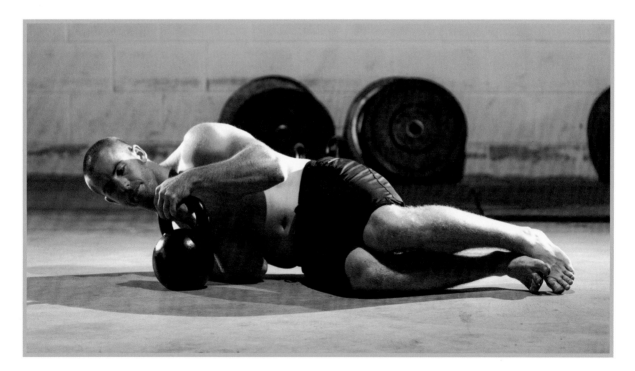

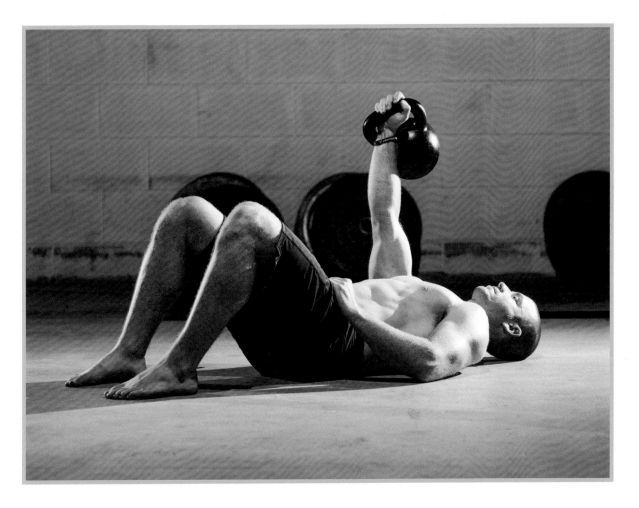

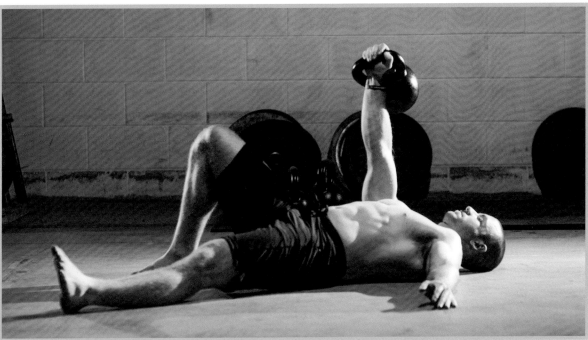

STEP 2: HAND AND FOOT SETUP

The client will pull their right foot in towards their body, making sure that the foot remains flat on the floor. The left arm should be straight, with the hand placed at a 45 degree angle from the shoulder. This important set up position will impact the remaining steps.

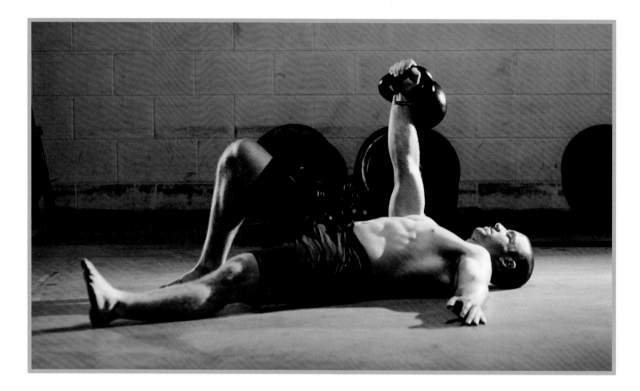

STEP 3: ROLL TO ELBOW

The emphasis of the movement should be a rotation from the spine, not lumbar forward flexion (as in a sit-up). To achieve the movement, the client should be instructed to push through the right foot and the elbow of the left arm to roll up to the elbow. Both shoulders should remain retracted and depressed throughout the movement. Watch for flexion in the thoracic spine, which will cause the shoulders to protract and elevate. Eyes should be fixed on the kettlebell.

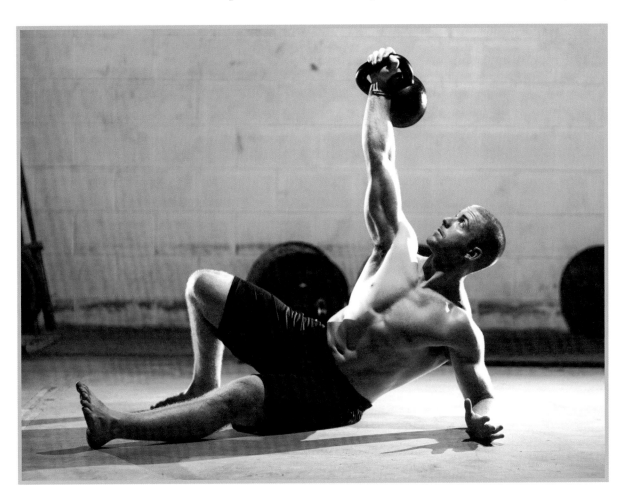

STEP 4: UP TO THE HAND

Maintaining the proper shoulder mechanics described in previous steps, press through the left hand to a locked out position. Rotate the hand so the fingers point behind. It is acceptable to adjust the left hand back and inward 3-5 inches to find a comfortable position. Watch out for the left shoulder protracting forward, giving the appearance of a "pointy" shoulder. Eyes should be on the kettlebell overhead.

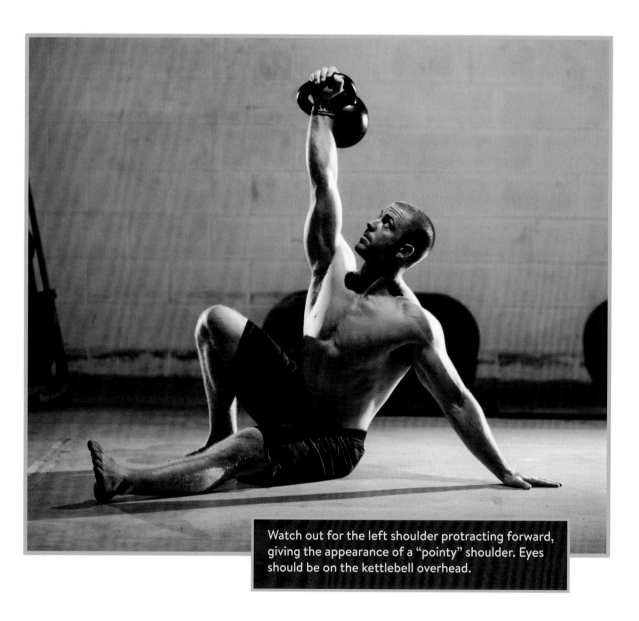

Watch out for the left shoulder protracting forward, giving the appearance of a "pointy" shoulder. Eyes should be on the kettlebell overhead.

STEP 5: HIGH BRIDGE

This next step is arguably one of the most important, because of its ability to open up the hips—which is desperately needed by most people. With the heel of the right foot remaining firmly on the ground, the client will push through the right heel while contracting the glute and extending the hips upward. Because the left lat connects through the thoracolumbar fascia to the opposite glute, you may cue the client to think of connecting their left lat to their right glute to improve the integrity of their high bridge. During the bridge, both shoulders should still remain retracted and depressed. The spine should be long including the neck, which can have a tendency to flex forward. Eyes should still be fixed on the kettlebell.

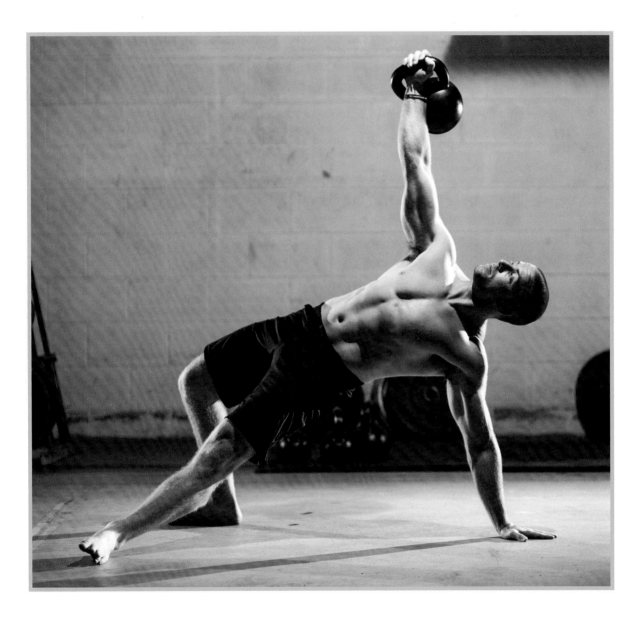

STEP 6: KNEE TO HAND

While maintaining pressure through the right heel, the client will smoothly slide their left knee to meet their left hand. This position can also be referred to as the "T" position since the arms and torso form a T shape. The spine should remain straight throughout the motion, with eyes on the kettlebell.

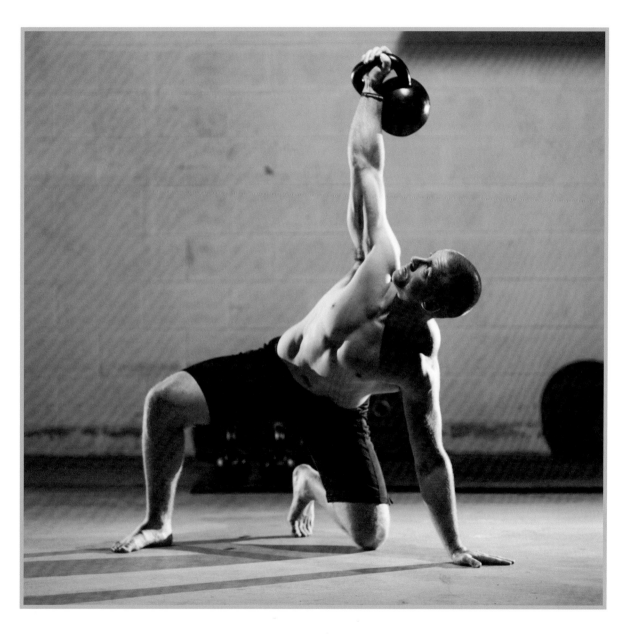

STEP 7: LUNGE

The next movement is driven by the left glute. The client will remove the left hand from the floor and bring the torso to vertical while maintaining a neutral spine. After a pause, the client will make sure both feet are parallel to each other. The pelvis shouldn't be tilted in a lateral, anterior, or posterior direction. Eyes are now looking straight ahead. There are two ways to align the feet. The first option is to pivot on the left knee until the feet are parallel. The second method is to rotate 90 degrees, bringing the right foot around until it is lined up. The second option is ideal for rough floor surfaces which prevent smooth pivoting on the knee, or if the client has a history of pressure-related knee pain.

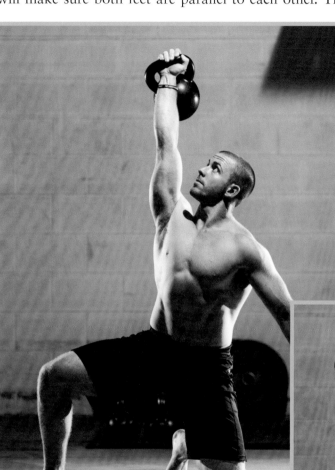

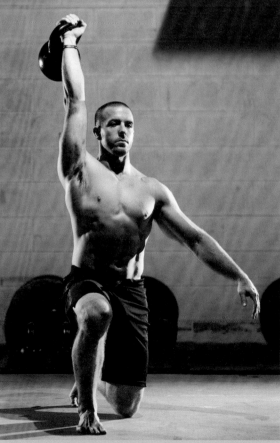

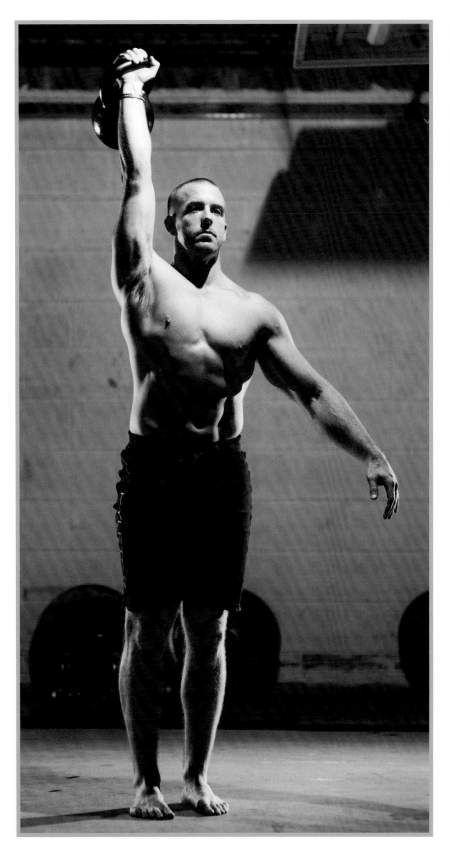

STEP 8: STAND

From a solid lunge position with the toes of the rear foot tucked under, drive through the front heel, contract the right glute and step forward to a standing position with feet together.

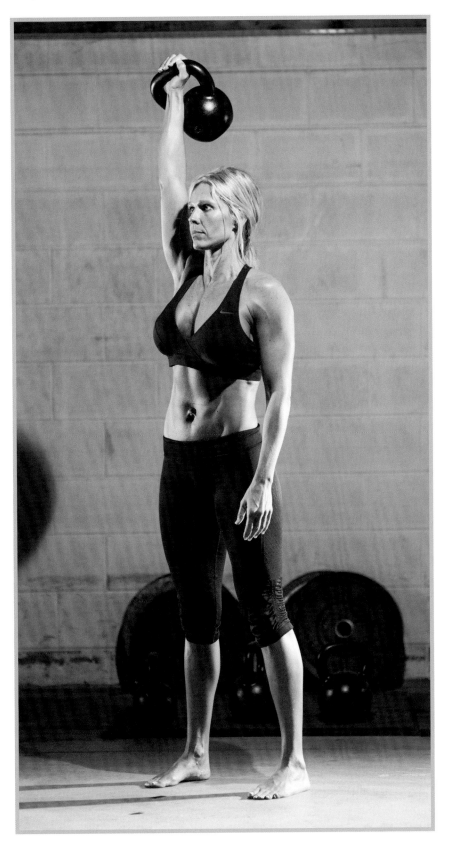

THE GET-UP STEPS IN REVERSE:

Reverse the motion, following each step in reverse until safely on the ground in the starting position. Eyes are facing straight ahead until the "T" position on the descent is reached.

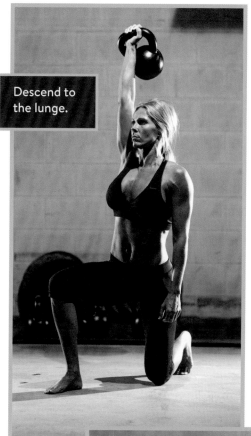

Descend to the lunge.

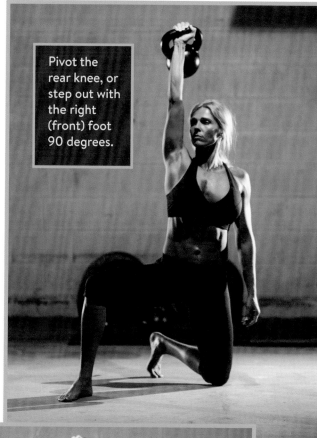

Pivot the rear knee, or step out with the right (front) foot 90 degrees.

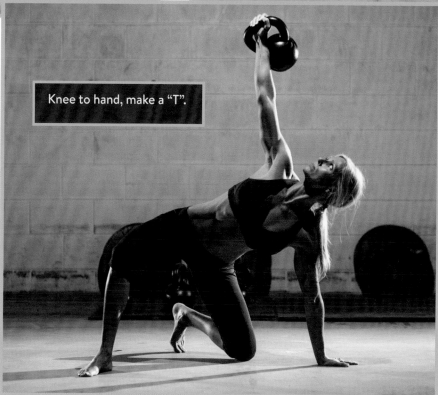

Knee to hand, make a "T".

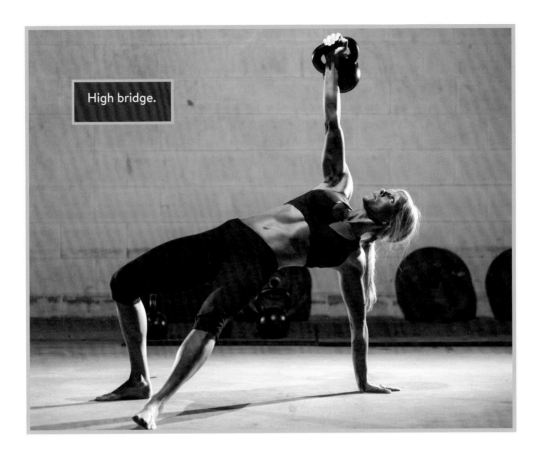

High bridge.

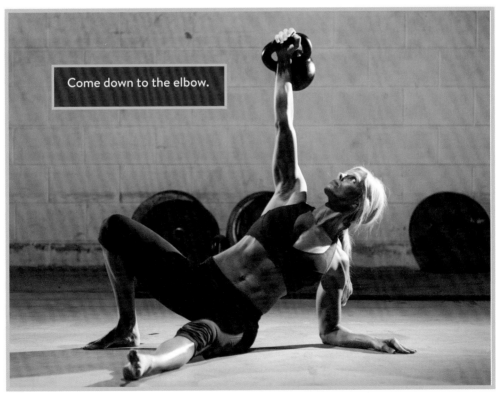

Come down to the elbow.

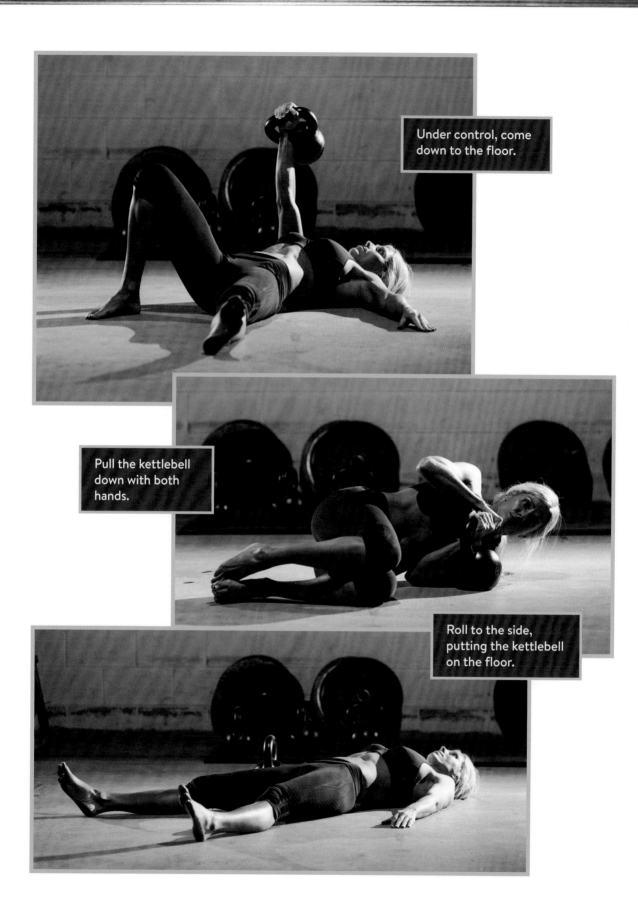

Under control, come down to the floor.

Pull the kettlebell down with both hands.

Roll to the side, putting the kettlebell on the floor.

It's important to teach the get-up in a safe environment. The client should perform unweighted get-ups until they are PERFECT before attempting it with a kettlebell. At first, the get-up will involve many awkward positions that might not feel comfortable, confident, or strong. The first rule when teaching the get-up is to ensure safety, and that means not using weight.

It is also a good idea to practice each step independently for repetitions. For example, a client could practice the roll to the elbow, or the high bridge 10 times in a row. It may be a good idea for some clients to simply practice the get-up as far as the high bridge if they lack the ability to stand up all the way due to strength or inflexibility. The get-up to high bridge is a terrific exercise on its own either for reps or held for time at the high bridge (like a plank).

IMPORTANT CUES FOR THE GET-UP:
- Shoulders down (away from ears)
- Long neck (to encourage proper shoulder position)
- Long spine
- Big chest (to ensure thoracic extension)

The get-up is an excellent drill that demands a lot of balance, coordination, and focus. The speed of the get-up should be similar to Tai Chi—methodical, purposeful, and moderate. There is no need to move especially slowly, but perfect control should be demonstrated during every second of the get-up. Never use an explosive burst to get through a difficult point in the get-up, or rush through the steps. Pause and own each position before proceeding.

GOBLET SQUAT

The goblet squat is the third foundational kettlebell exercise. The squat is arguably the most fundamental human movement pattern—and it's still a resting position in countries where chairs are not readily available. A properly performed squat requires adequate mobility in the ankles, hips, and knees. Humans are born able to squat comfortably and easily, but the ability is often lost with a sedentary, unnatural lifestyle. The "use it or lose it" principle applies to the squat movement pattern. From an exercise standpoint, the squat is an amazing lower body strengthening exercise that requires stability through the midsection along with strength and flexibility throughout the legs and hips. The goblet squat is the best way to teach good movement patterns in the squat using a kettlebell.

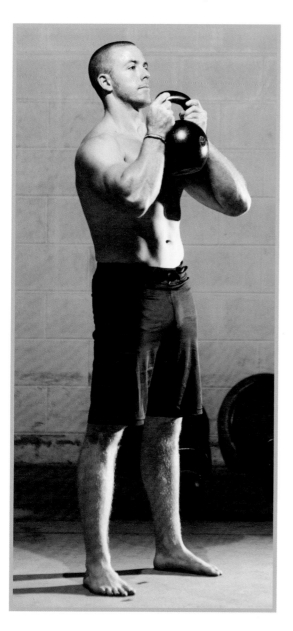

To begin, have the client grasp the kettlebell by the horns (sides of handle) while holding it up to their chest. Instruct the client to "sit back" instead of dropping down. At the bottom position, they should touch their elbows to the inside of their knees (vastus medialis). The resulting position will look like this:

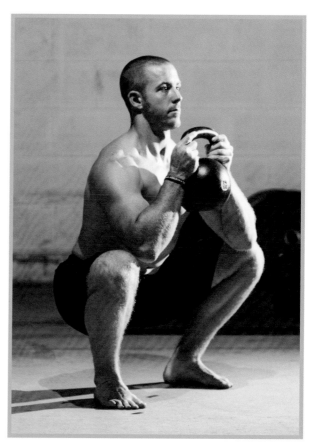

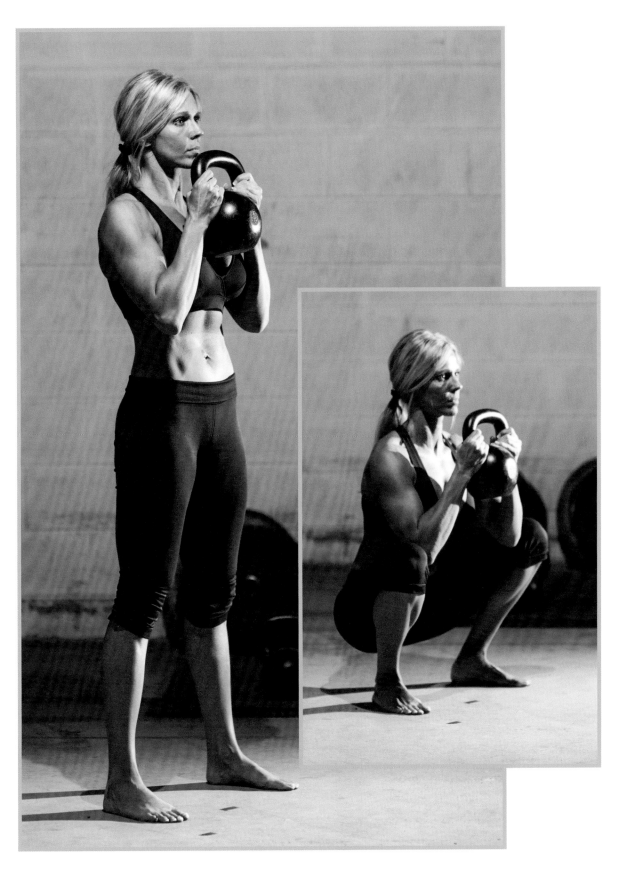

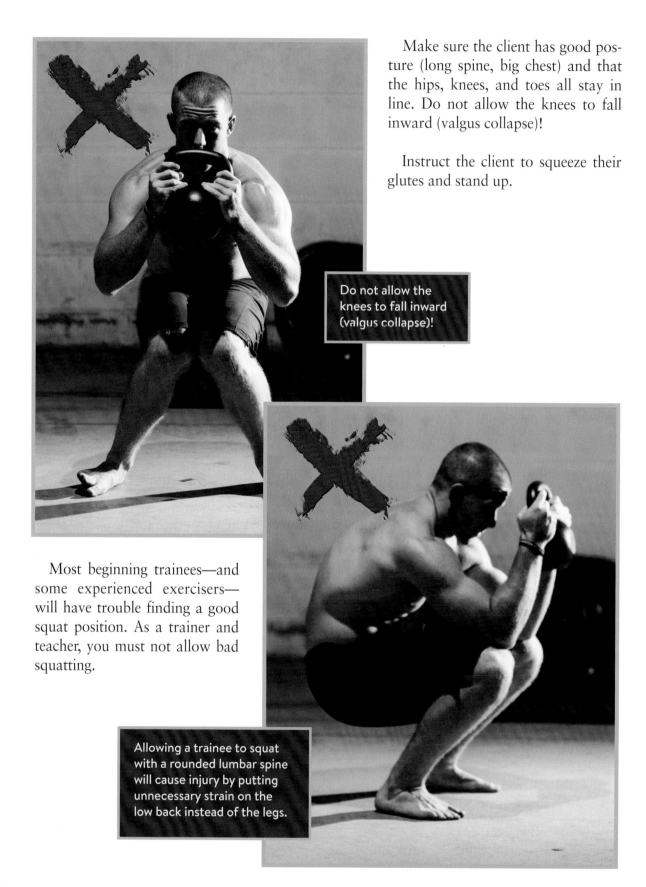

Make sure the client has good posture (long spine, big chest) and that the hips, knees, and toes all stay in line. Do not allow the knees to fall inward (valgus collapse)!

Instruct the client to squeeze their glutes and stand up.

Do not allow the knees to fall inward (valgus collapse)!

Most beginning trainees—and some experienced exercisers—will have trouble finding a good squat position. As a trainer and teacher, you must not allow bad squatting.

Allowing a trainee to squat with a rounded lumbar spine will cause injury by putting unnecessary strain on the low back instead of the legs.

Apart from being a great strength exercise, the squat is a good way to increase flexibility in the hips and ankles. Starting in the bottom position of a squat, have the client use their elbows to push outward on the knees to open up the hips. Next, have the client shift their weight side-to-side, further opening up the hips. This stretching concept—"prying"—is attributed to Pavel Tsatsouline. Once the hip mobilization drill is complete, the client may set the bell down before standing up.

IMPORTANT CUES FOR THE GOBLET SQUAT:

- Big chest
- Long spine
- Hips, knees, and toes are on the same line
- Weight is evenly distributed through feet, heels must push through the floor and not come up
- Spine does not round during movement
- Sit back rather than fall down

The goblet squat is a very valuable tool for putting together a complete strength and conditioning program using kettlebells. Don't dismiss the goblet squat as movement only for "beginners". Continue to refine and add weight to it when appropriate. When combined with the swing, the squat will help achieve a balance between hip (hinging in the swing) and knee dominant (goblet squat) leg exercises. This will ensure balance between the front and back musculature of the leg, making the client more resistant to injury.

The goblet squat, swing, and get-up demonstrate many positive movement qualities. The get-up involves lifting an asymmetrical load through various ranges of motion at the shoulder joint, and an asymmetrical lower body strength movement (lunge). The swing provides a symmetrical hip-hinge, core stability, and hip extension. The goblet squat requires a symmetrical stance, stability thorough the core (abdomen), and flexibility and strength of the lower body. When clients achieve competency in these three movements, they will be more mobile, flexible, strong, and resistant to injury.

KETTLEBELL CLEAN

The clean movement is built from a good swing. Do not attempt to teach the clean to a client who is not competent with safe kettlebell swings.

The clean is the best method for bringing one or two kettlebells to the rack position. In the rack position, the kettlebell is held at the chest with the bell resting on the forearm and the wrist straight.

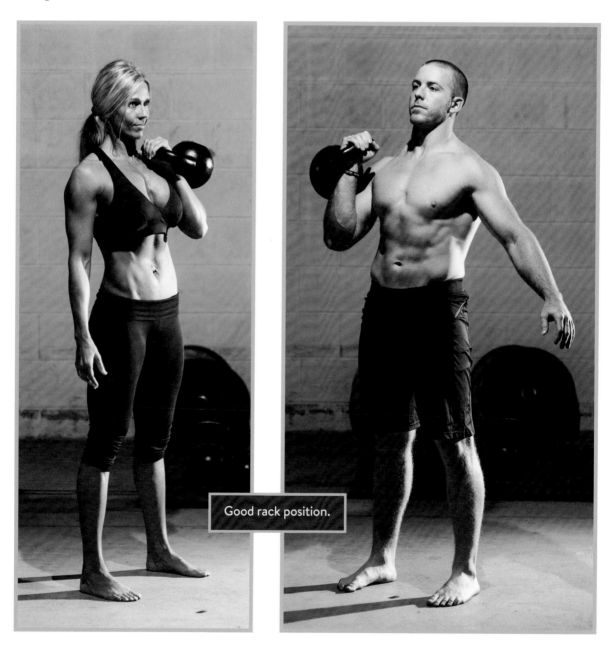

Good rack position.

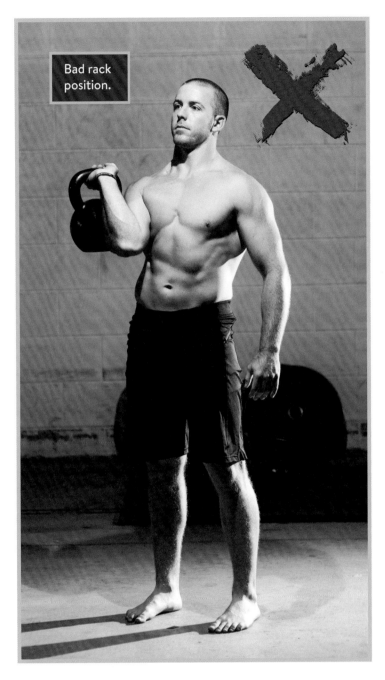

Bad rack position.

When holding kettlebells in the rack position, keep legs straight and don't lean backwards. Stand up tall!

To begin the clean, swing the bell back between the legs just as you did with the swing. This time, instead of keeping the palm facing backwards, slightly internally rotate, pointing the thumb's side of the handle backwards. This will engage and strengthen the rotator cuff during the ascent of the bell(s). After the backswing, simply extend the hips and knees as in the swing, and slightly pull back on the bell to pop it up so it rotates around the forearm and lands safely in the rack position. A loose grip is necessary for the bell to rotate in the hand. Finish the movement by shooting the hand upward through the handle instead of the bell crashing down.

A good cue for the clean is to point back with the thumb during the back swing, then point to the clavicle in the top position.

The client should learn to hold the kettlebell comfortably in the rack position while walking.

Dropping the kettlebell from the clean should simply be the reverse of the racking movement—the client will let the bell rotate around the arm and fall back into the same groove as the swing. After it drops into a swing position, the kettlebell follows the same backswing between the legs. The client should be able to perform multiple cleans in succession without setting the bell down. One advantage the kettlebell has over a barbell is multiple reps of the swing, clean, or snatch can be performed continuously without the need to stop and reset. This advantage allows for fluid movement and greater safety during high rep exercise sessions.

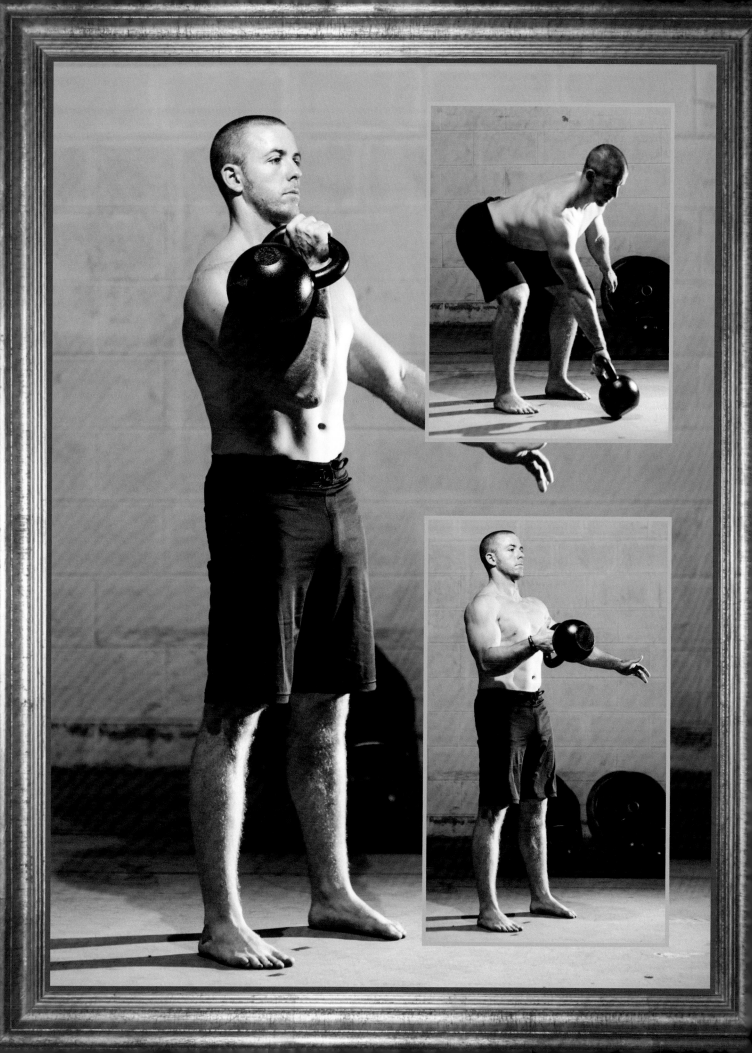

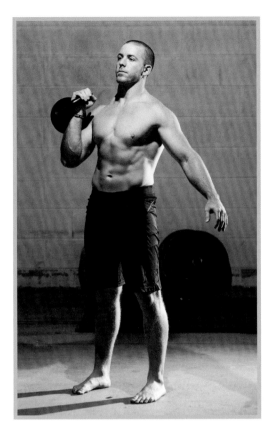

THE PRESS

The most highly regarded upper body movement is the kettlebell military press. The kettlebell military press differs from a standard dumbbell press because the kettlebell allows for a larger range of motion and has a displaced center of gravity. This displacement also requires greater strength and coordination from the user. To have a good press, one must already have a strong get-up. Clients proficient in the get-up will have the shoulder mobility and stability required to work with a kettlebell overhead. The press starts where the clean ends—the rack position. From the rack position, press the kettlebell up and out to the side, ending in a solid overhead position while keeping the scapula depressed. Never let the shoulder blade elevate during the press, this creates instability and can cause injury to the shoulder.

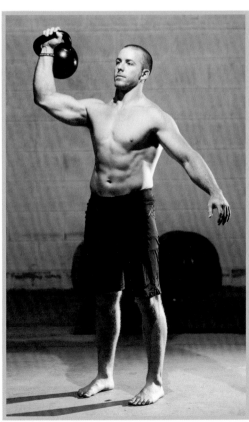

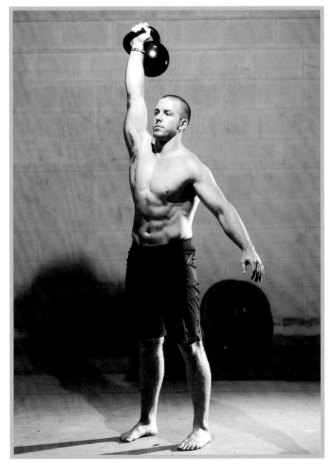

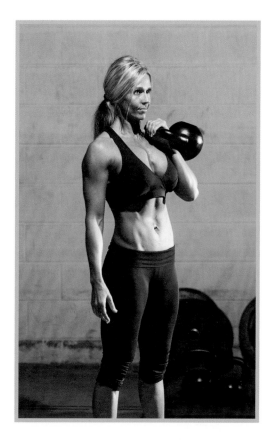

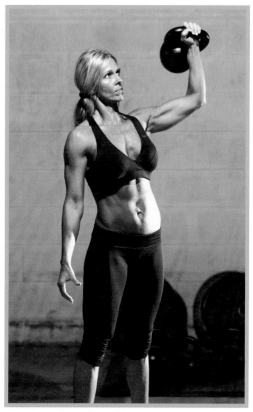

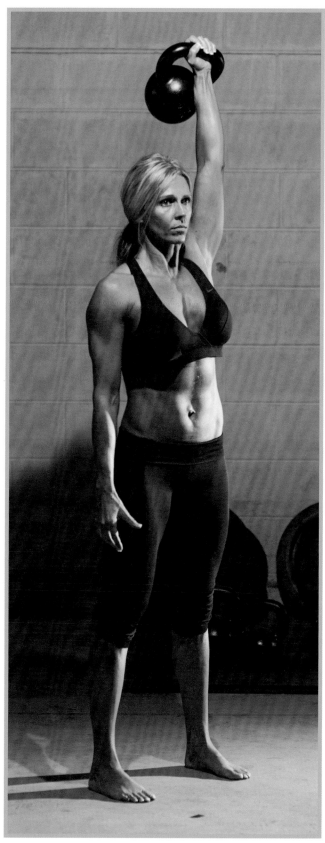

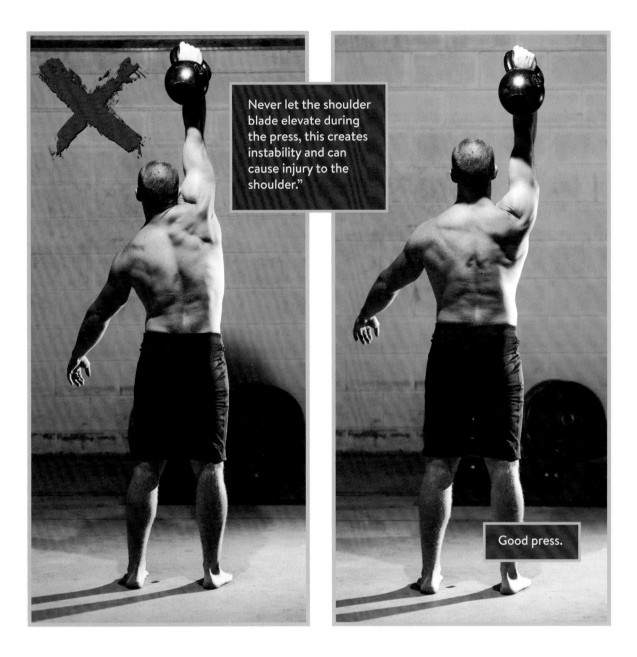

Never let the shoulder blade elevate during the press, this creates instability and can cause injury to the shoulder."

Good press.

IMPORTANT CUES FOR THE PRESS:
- Forearm stays vertical
- Wrist stays straight
- Posture remains tall
- Scapula is depressed and retracted into the socket

After mastering the one arm press, the press can be performed with both arms:

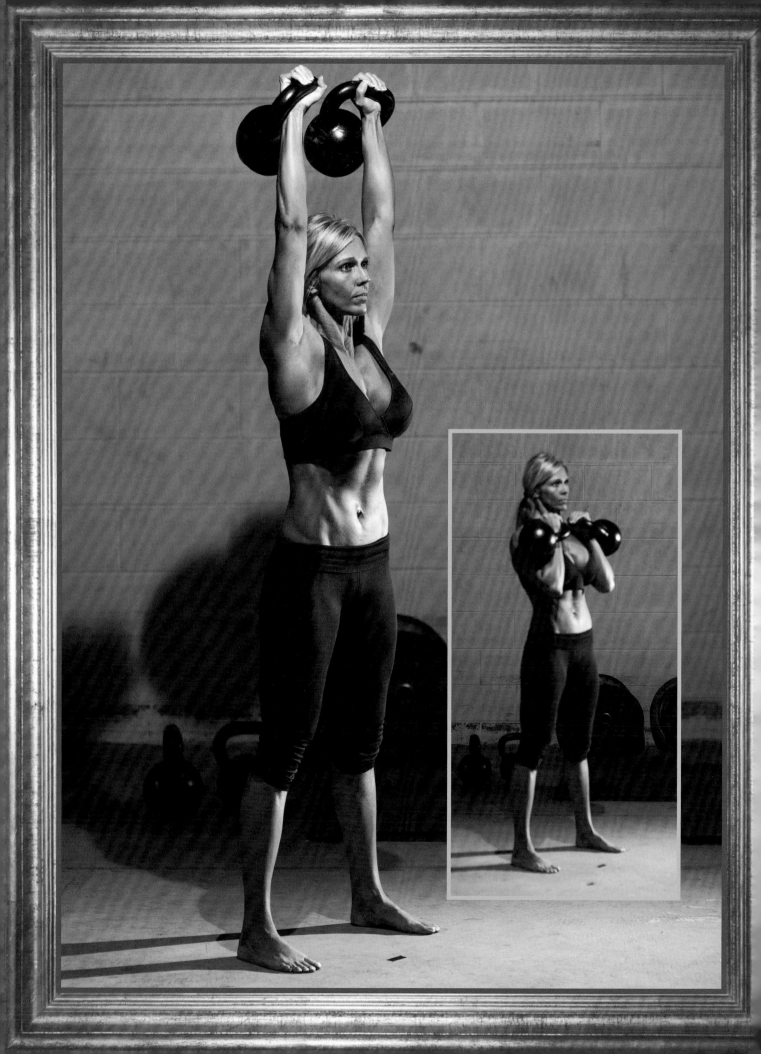

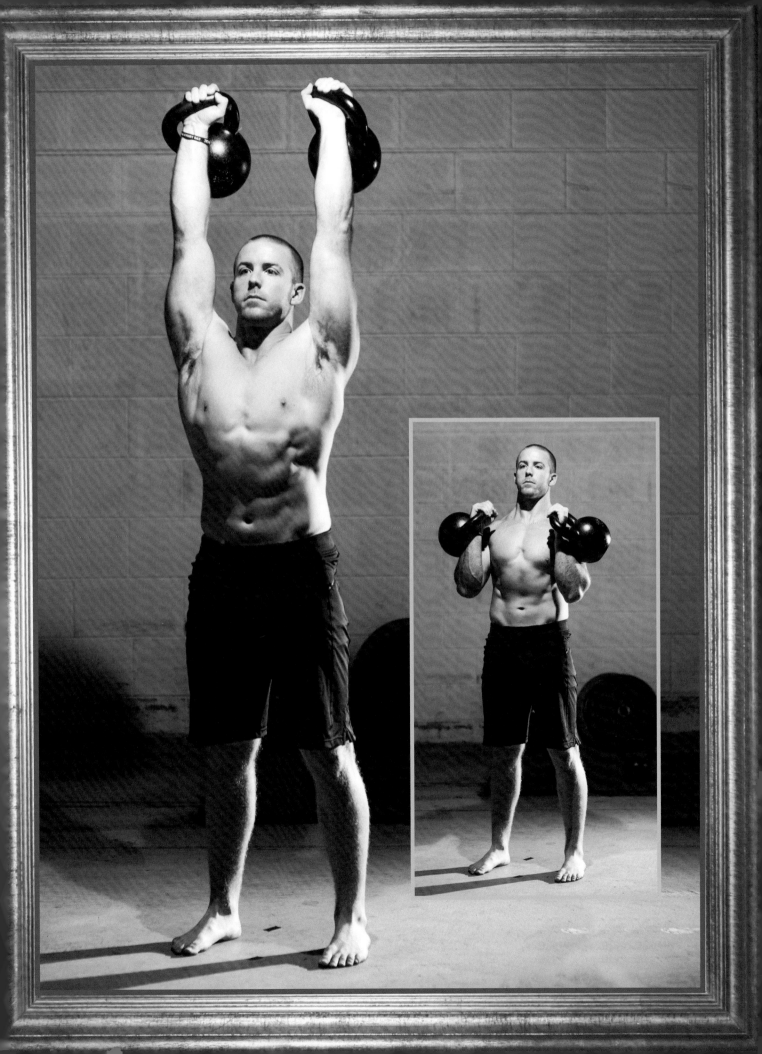

BOTTOM UP PRESS

The bottom up press is a military press variation that offers many benefits and is completely unique to kettlebell training. I recommend that the bottom up press be the PRIMARY upper body pushing exercise with kettlebells. You will find that with the bottom up press the cues from the standard military press happen automatically, making it great for learning the movement properly. Along with single arm swings, the bottom up press is one of my two favorite kettlebell movements.

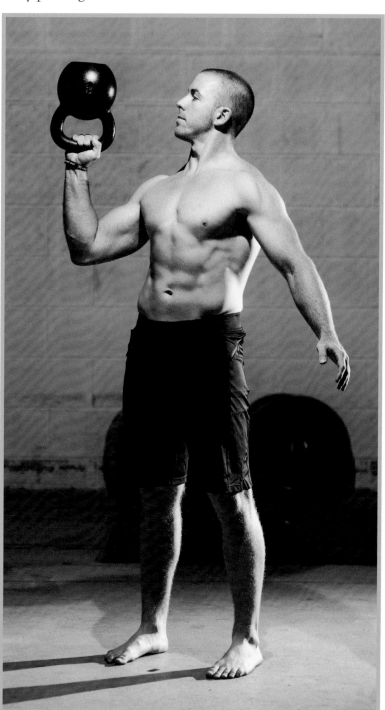

The bottom up press requires shoulder stability, balance, coordination, grip strength, and stability through the torso and lower body. This difficult press variation can be used to correct problems some people may have with the standard military press, such as keeping the forearm vertical or letting the shoulder pop out of the socket.

To begin, grasp the kettlebell on the floor and push your weight into the handle as if you were going to do a push-up.

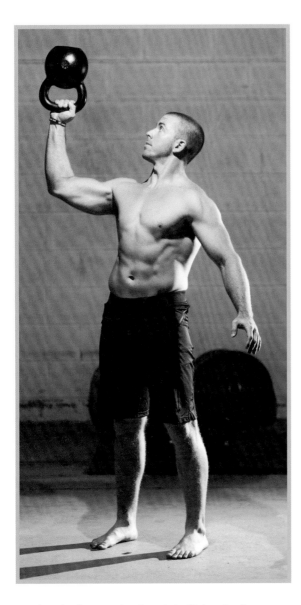

Maintain this crushing grip as you bring the kettlebell up to the shoulder, balancing it upside down.

From this position, keep your eyes on the bell and press the weight overhead as in the standard press.

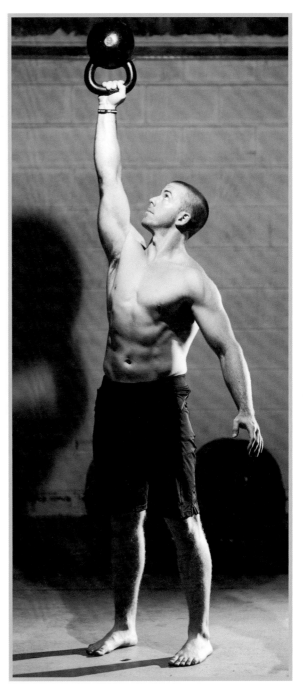

Slowly bring the kettlebell back down to the shoulder for the next press, or set it down safely by using a normal backswing.

The bottom up press is a very demanding drill that requires strength and focus. Practice this drill sparingly to avoid burnout and keep the reps low (1-5) for the best results.

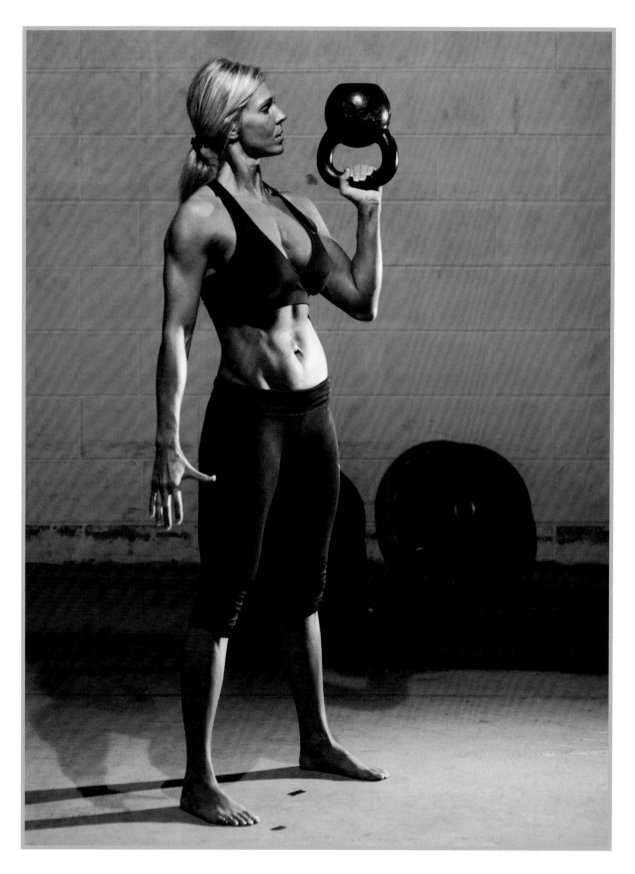

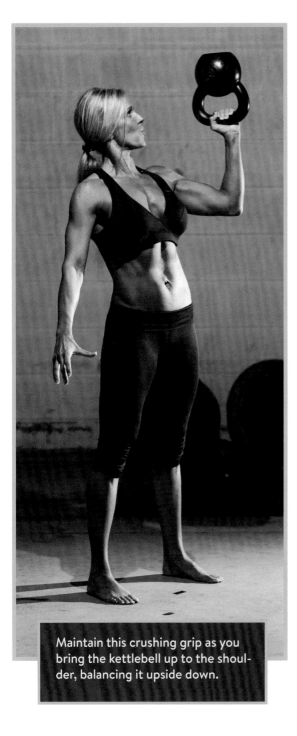

Maintain this crushing grip as you bring the kettlebell up to the shoulder, balancing it upside down.

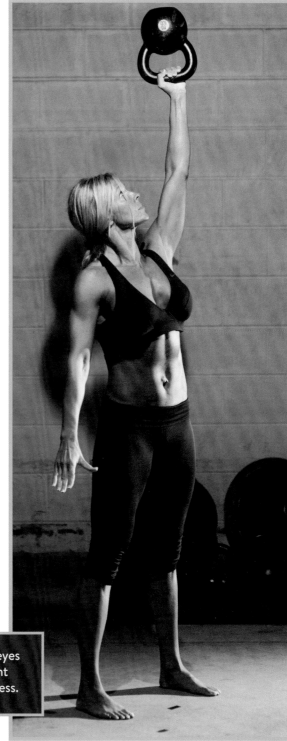

From this position, keep your eyes on the bell and press the weight overhead as in the standard press.

THE SNATCH

The kettlebell snatch is risky for the average user. It demands a very strong and stable shoulder girdle, and a lot of high speed coordination. A kettlebell snatch is similar to a swing, but ends with the kettlebell overhead.

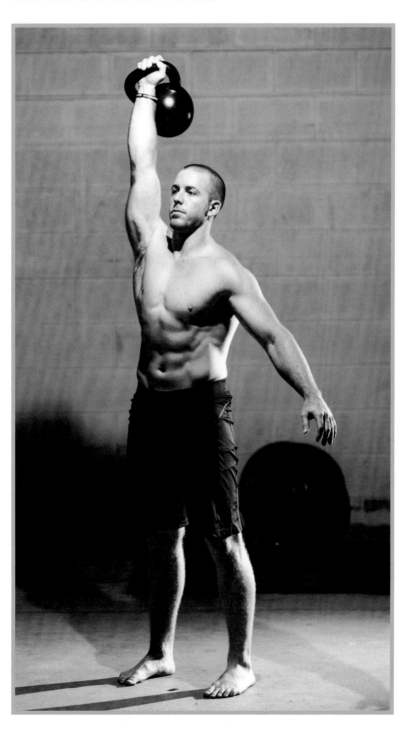

Do not attempt the snatch until the swing is mastered. No good can come from rushing to learn the kettlebell snatch. The swing is the foundation of kettlebell training for a reason, and should be practiced accordingly. Even though the snatch is more technically difficult, it should not be considered an "advanced" swing. But, note how the first half of the snatch is identical to the swing:

Where the snatch differs is the second half of the movement. The trajectory of the kettlebell changes when the weight is pulled into the body. The energy is no longer projected forward, it's moving upward instead.

Once the kettlebell reaches eye level, think of punching the ceiling while spearing your hand through the handle (as if you were putting on a glove). This will ensure that the bell doesn't flip over at the top with so much force that it crashes into the wrist and forearm.

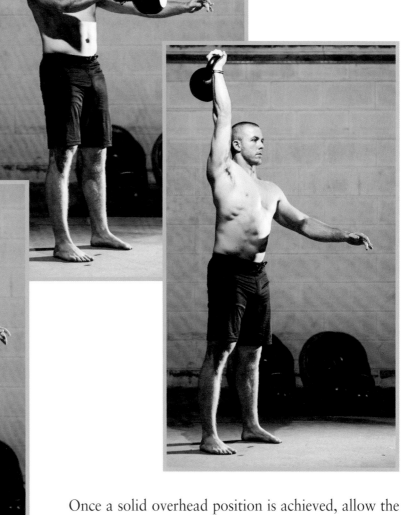

Once a solid overhead position is achieved, allow the bell to spin around the forearm as it descends. This will feel similar to the descent of the kettlebell during the clean. Re-grip the handle with your fingers and repeat the exercise with a normal backswing.

IMPORTANT CUES FOR SNATCHES:

- The shoulder must stay in the socket. The elbow and wrist are straight at the top position.
- Just like the swing, the power should come from the hips. If the client uses their arms too much, revisit swings again before progressing with snatches.
- Snatches can be very taxing on the hands, be wary of blisters and tears while doing snatches.

The average gym user, and even a fit person does not need to add snatches to their kettlebell training. The potential risk involved is generally not worth the minimal reward. All things being equal, it is recommended to diligently train the swing rather than perform kettlebell snatches.

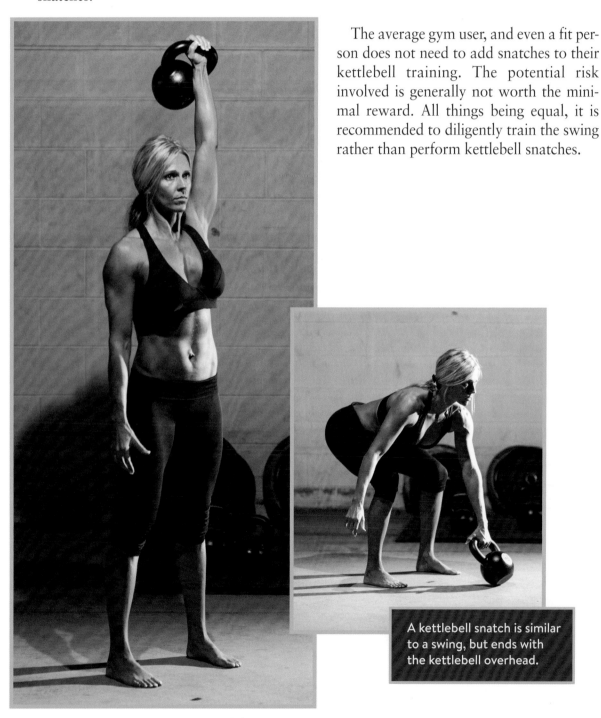

A kettlebell snatch is similar to a swing, but ends with the kettlebell overhead.

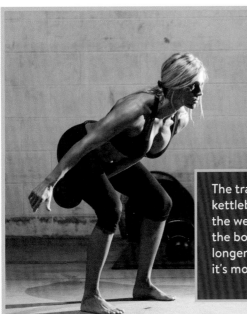

The trajectory of the kettlebell changes when the weight is pulled into the body. The energy is no longer projected forward, it's moving upward instead.

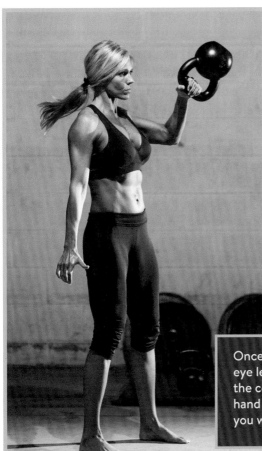

Once the kettlebell reaches eye level, think of punching the ceiling while spearing your hand through the handle (as if you were putting on a glove).

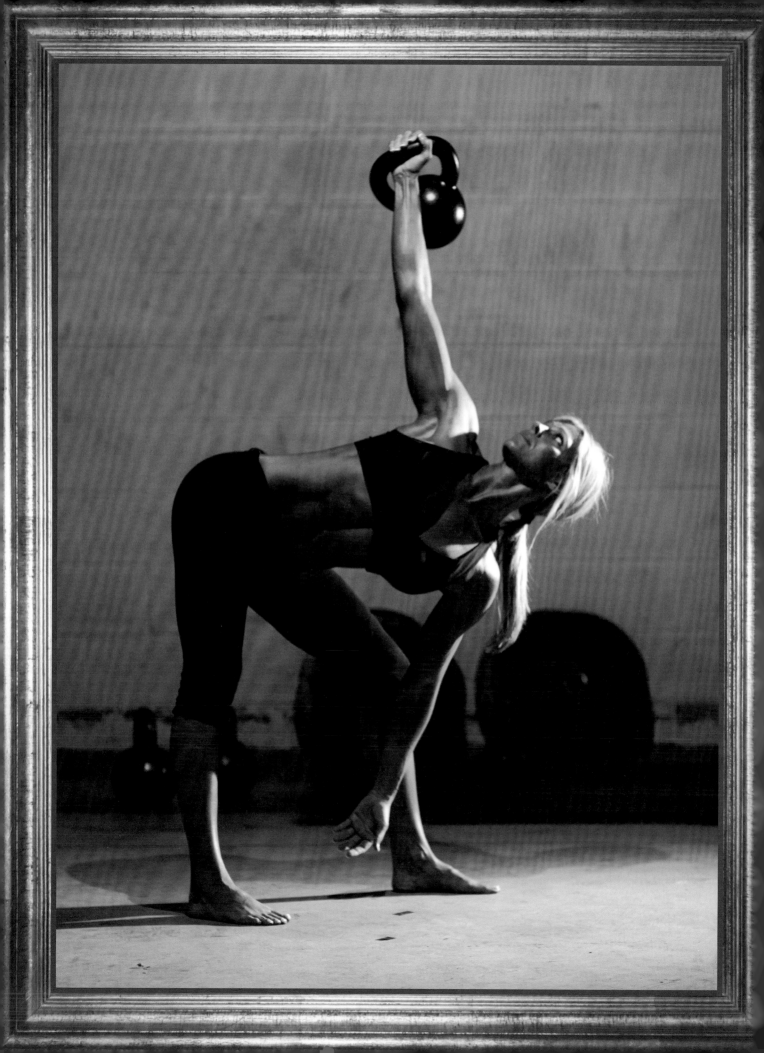

CHAPTER FOUR

KETTLEBELL SPECIFIC EXERCISES

The design of the kettlebell provides unique benefits and allows for exercises above and beyond traditional weights. The following section contains exercises that are either unique to kettlebells or are traditionally associated with kettlebell training.

THE WINDMILL

The Windmill is an exercise commonly associated with kettlebell training.

To perform the windmill, begin by pressing a kettlebell overhead. Stand with both feet at a 45 degree angle, pointed away from the arm with the kettlebell. For example, if the kettlebell is held in the right hand, the feet will be pointed towards the left.

Next, hip hinge by pushing your hips away from your feet, just as you would in a swing. Be sure to hinge towards the side with the kettlebell. If the kettlebell is held in the right hand, your hips will push back towards the right. As you hinge, slide the back of your free hand along the inside of your front leg. Keep your eyes on the kettlebell at all times!

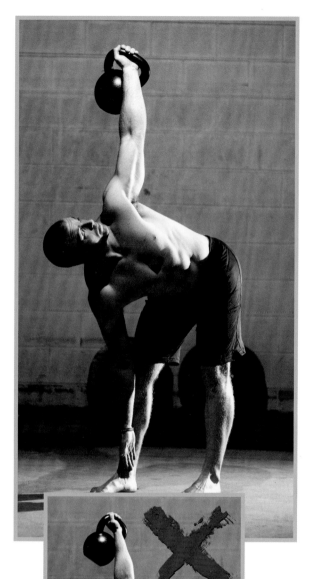

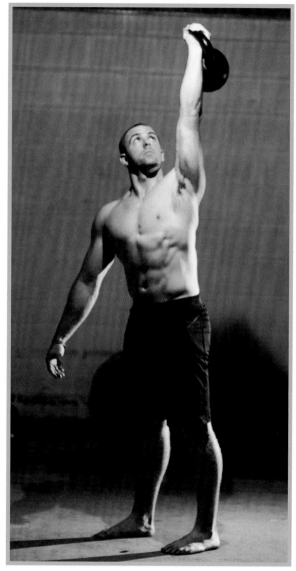

Once you have reached the end of your flexibility, return to the start position by squeezing the glutes and standing up.

Note: Like a deadlift or swing, the windmill demands a strict hip hinge with no forward flexion at the spine. The downward movement should come from the hips while the spine rotates to open up the chest.

Bad windmill.

When properly executed, the windmill is a terrific exercise for shoulder stability and flexibility of the thoracic spine and hips. It also requires a strong core, and specifically targets the obliques. The windmill is best learned without weight so that this challenging movement can be smoothly coordinated.

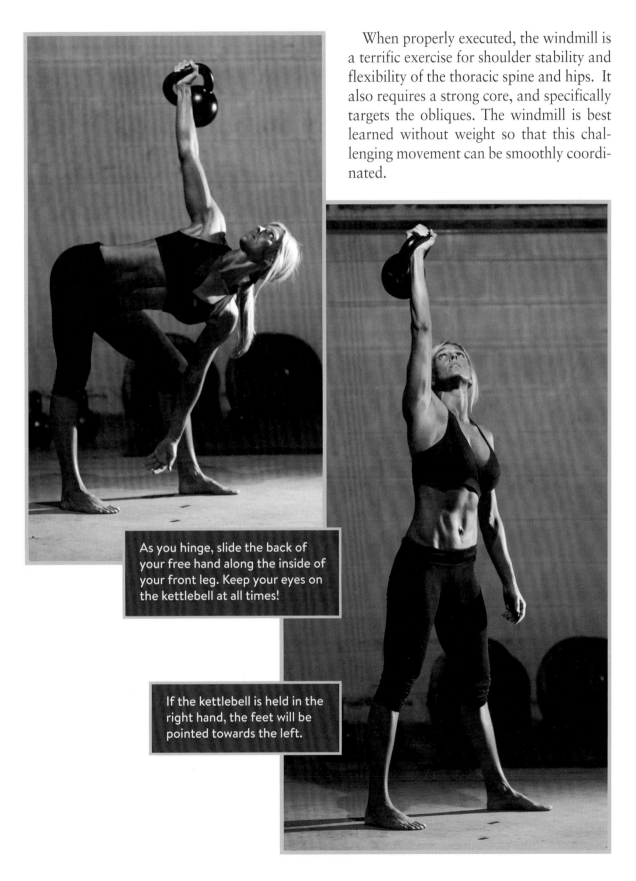

As you hinge, slide the back of your free hand along the inside of your front leg. Keep your eyes on the kettlebell at all times!

If the kettlebell is held in the right hand, the feet will be pointed towards the left.

KETTLEBELL PASSING DRILLS

The offset handle on a kettlebell makes it easy to pass the bell back and forth between hands. Here are a few maneuvers which take advantage of the kettlebell's unique design.

AROUND THE WORLD

The kettlebell is passed around the body while the torso remains forward. Pass the kettlebell in front and behind the body with a clean hand-off. This drill can be used as an effective warm up, a grip challenge, and a core exercise. Be careful not to compromise good form by choosing a kettlebell that's too heavy . Be sure to brace the midsection to keep it stable, and to avoid moving from the spine in this drill. Make sure to stay balanced by performing the drill in both directions.

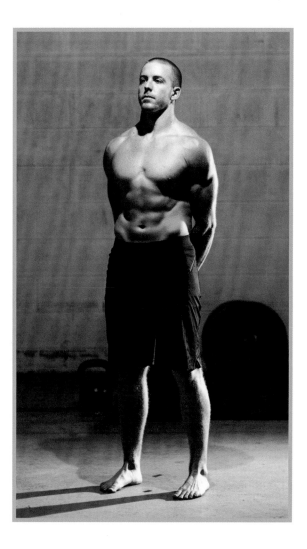
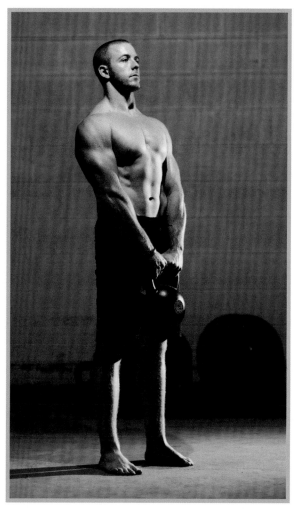

FIGURE 8 TO A HOLD

The figure 8 to a hold involves passing a kettlebell between the legs using a swing motion. Begin by performing a standard one arm swing. On the downswing, angle the bell slightly away from the working arm and pass the bell between the legs to the opposite hand. Once the bell is in the opposite hand, stand up as in the standard swing and bring the ball of the kettlebell to the opposite palm. Hold this position. The abs should be braced and the spine should never go into forward flexion. From the hold, swing the kettlebell back and repeat the movement on the other side.

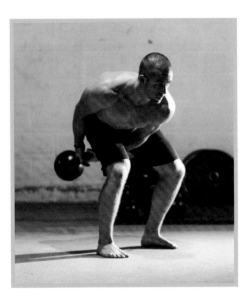
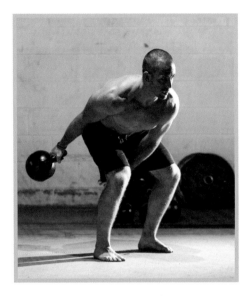
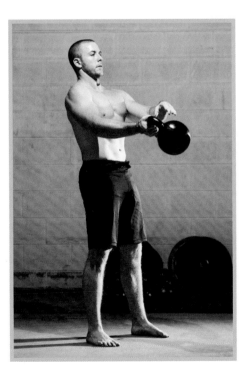
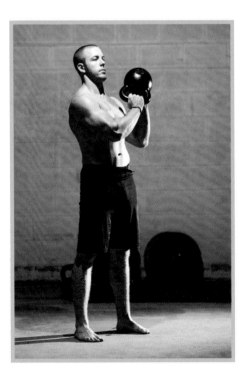

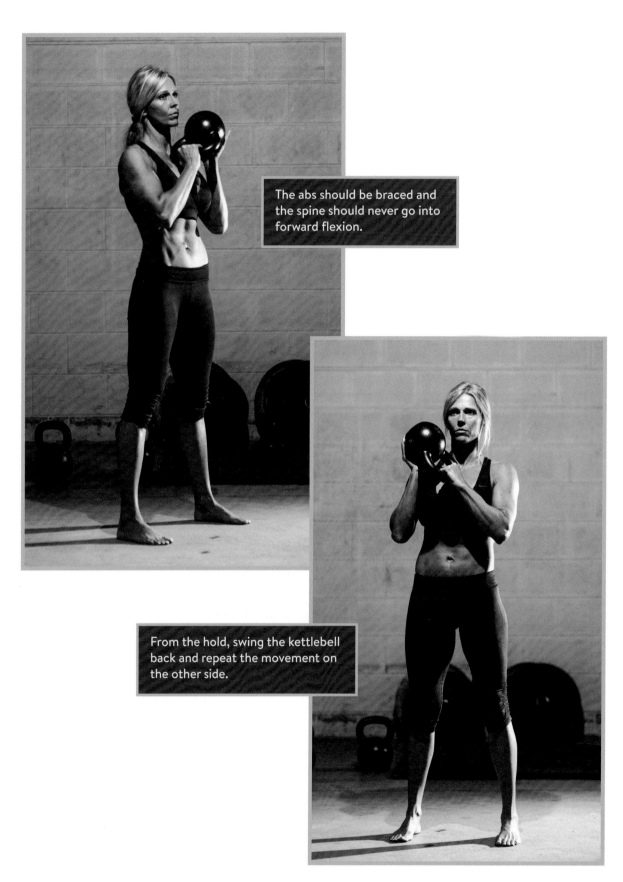

The abs should be braced and the spine should never go into forward flexion.

From the hold, swing the kettlebell back and repeat the movement on the other side.

KETTLEBELL JUGGLING

Kettlebell juggling requires a lot of coordination, grip strength, and a solid swing. Because of the interest in juggling kettlebells, we have included a brief introduction, but please note that this is not a comprehensive guide to juggling.

STANDARD FLIP

The standard flip should be the starting point for anyone interested in juggling kettlebells.

Begin by swinging the kettlebell with both hands. At the apex of the swing—slightly above chest level—let go of the bell, letting it float momentarily before re-gripping and swinging it back again. Once you feel comfortable floating the kettlebell at the apex of the swing, flip the bell upward by flicking the wrists into extension. After the handle makes a full revolution, re-grip the bell and continue into a standard downswing. The standard flip can be practiced with one or two hands, and with one or two kettlebells. Kettlebells can also be flipped sideways, and the standard flip can be applied to moves like the figure 8 (flip instead of hold). However, it is absolutely imperative to have a solid mastery of the standard swing before attempting any kettlebell juggling. That being said, kettlebell juggling can be a great method to keep training mentally stimulating and fun.

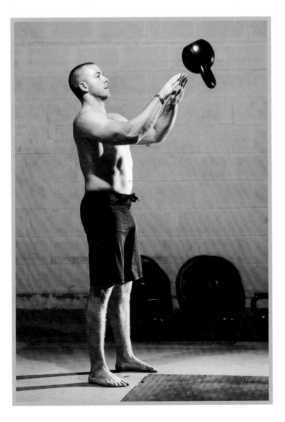 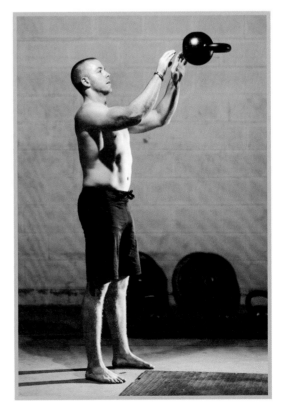

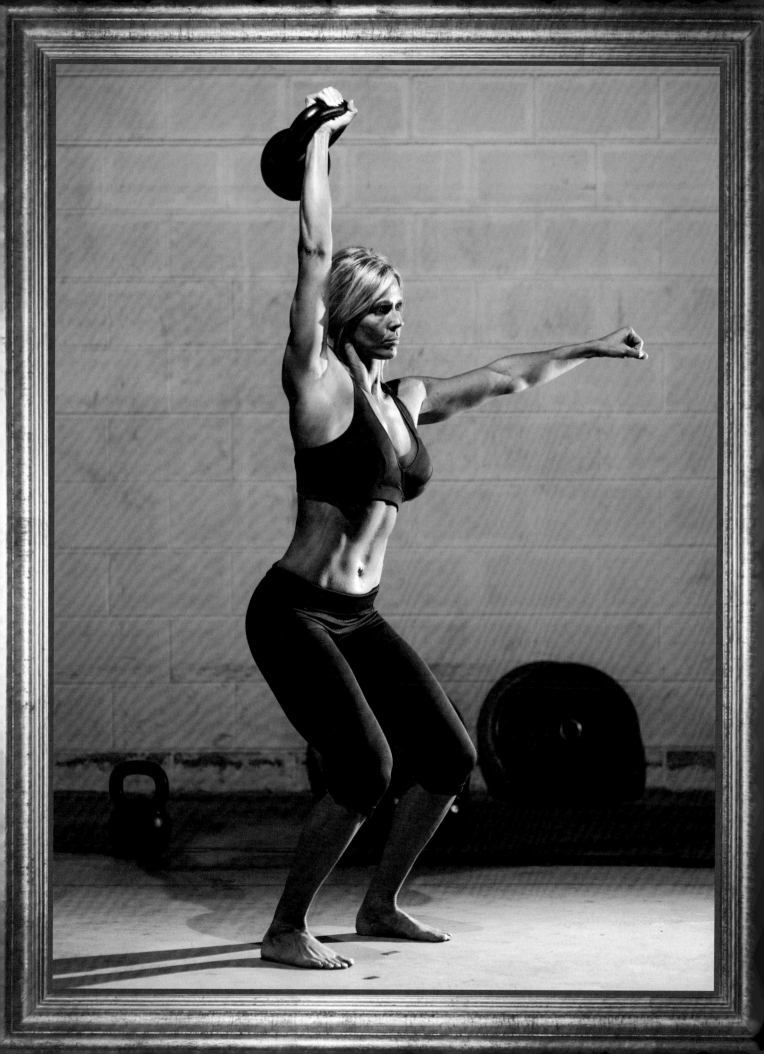

CHAPTER FIVE

BASIC PLANES OF MOTION

O ur approach to exercise focuses on movements instead of individual muscles. But, with a good understanding of the basic planes of motion involved in the exercises, the muscles involved in the movement patterns will become obvious. For the sake of simplicity, the main movements will be split into upper pushing and pulling, and lower pushing and pulling. Upper body movements will be further categorized within the vertical and horizontal planes. Lower body movements will be classified as either hip-dominant or knee-dominant. Bilateral and unilateral movements will also be included for the upper and lower body.

By categorizing these exercises, it's easier to craft an appropriately balanced training program. This is especially important concerning upper body training. It's all too common for exercise programs to be overly focused on pushing. This can cause serious problems with postural alignment and shoulder health. When a program focuses too much on pushing in the horizontal plane (for example with the bench press) without a balance of horizontal pulling exercises, the pecs and biceps tighten and shorten, protracting the scapula forward. This exacerbates the common but dysfunctional postural alignment (forward flexed kyphotic posture) explained in the introduction. This imbalance between the front and back of the body is a common cause of shoulder pain and impingement, resulting in a loss of ROM and poor performance.

A balanced approach is also important for lower body exercises. Most clients will start with sensory-motor amnesia of the glutes coupled with tight, short, and weak hip flexors. These clients will be quad-dominant during exercise and in their daily lives. An imbalance between the front and back of the leg is a major cause of knee pain and ultimately back pain when the quadratus lumborum is overused to compensate for a lack of hip extension. It is very important to balance exercises involving the front and back of the thigh (hamstrings and gluteal muscles vs quadriceps and hip flexors), and to achieve synergy between them. In order for a program to have balance, there must be balance between movements.

- Horizontal pushing must be balanced with horizontal pulling.
- Vertical pushing must be balanced with vertical pulling.
- Knee dominant leg exercises must be balanced with hip dominant leg exercises.

To assist in creating a complete, balanced program, the following pages are an exercise index organized by movement category rather than specific muscles.

UPPER BODY:
VERTICAL PUSHING:
BILATERAL:

MILITARY PRESS

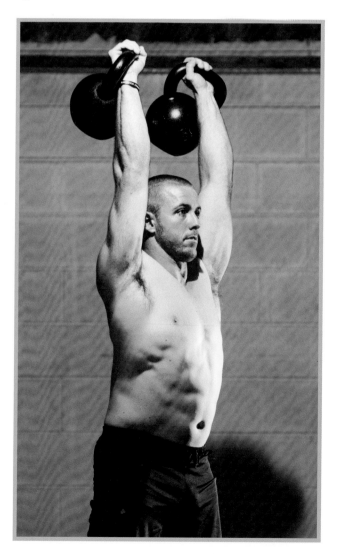

PUSH PRESS

Begin with two kettlebells in the rack position. Drop into a slight squat and drive the bells overhead using momentum from the legs. Finish the lockout with the shoulders and triceps. End at a full standing position.

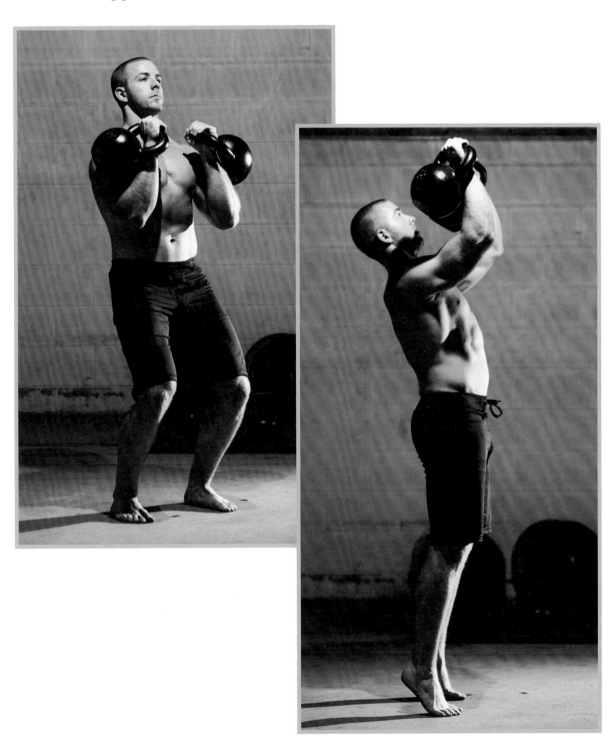

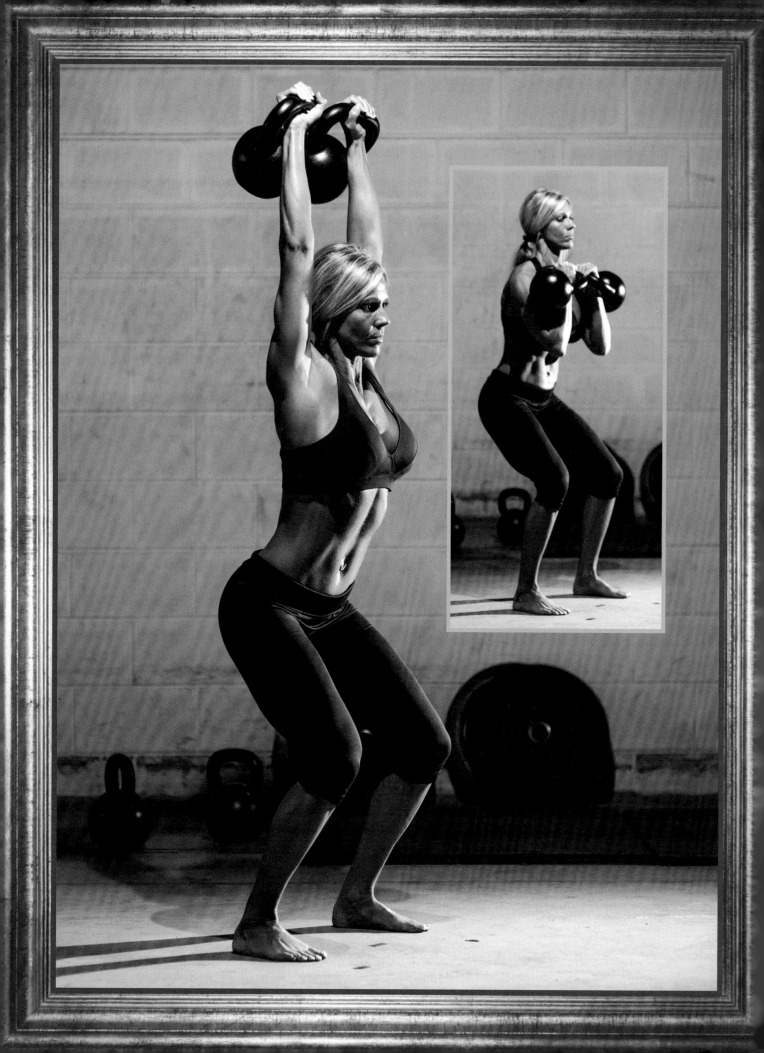

JERK

Begin with two kettlebells in the rack position. Drop into a slight squat and drive the bells upward by jumping up explosively. Land in a shallow squat stance with both arms locked out overhead. Stand up to finish.

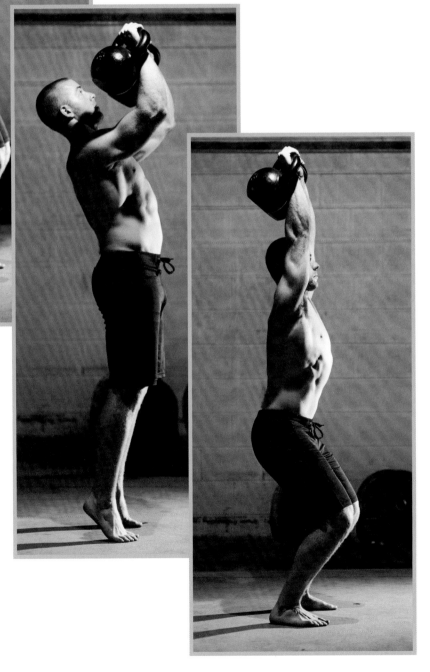

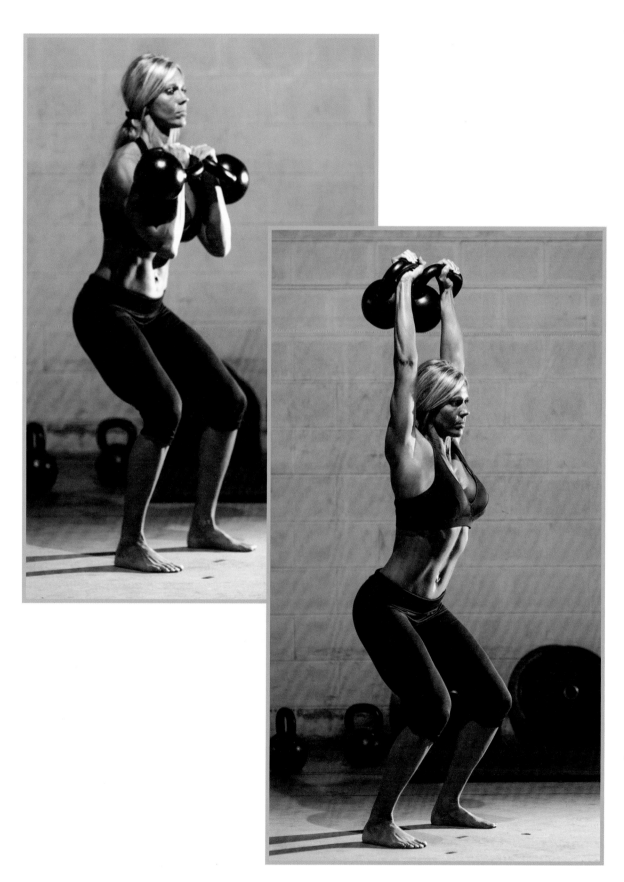

UNILATERAL:

ONE ARM MILITARY PRESS

See Exercises section for detailed description.

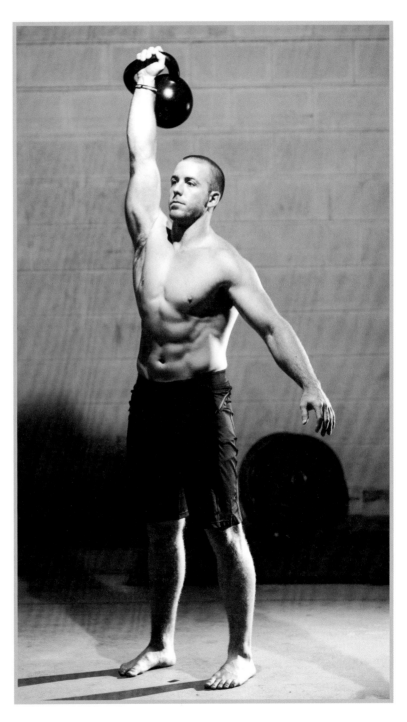

ONE ARM PUSH PRESS

Begin with one kettlebell in the rack position. Drop into a slight squat and drive the bell overhead using momentum from the legs. Finish the lockout with the shoulder and triceps, and end at a full standing position.

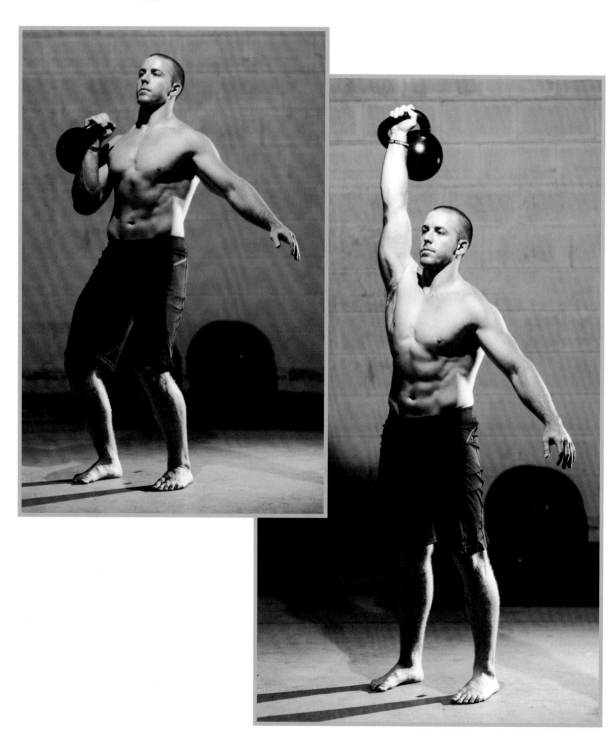

ONE ARM JERK

Begin with one kettlebell in the rack position. Drop into a slight squat and drive the bell upward by jumping up explosively. Land in a shallow squat stance with the arm holding the kettlebell locked out overhead. Stand up to finish.

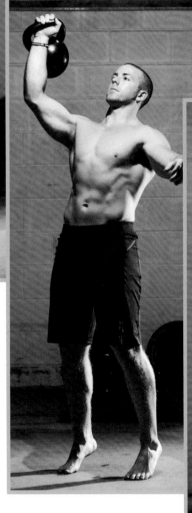

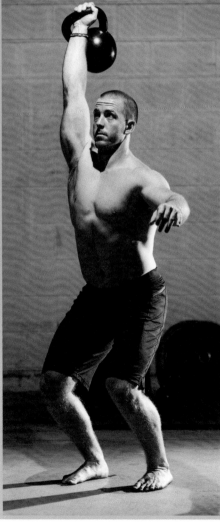

BOTTOM UP PRESS

See Exercise section on the press for a detailed description.

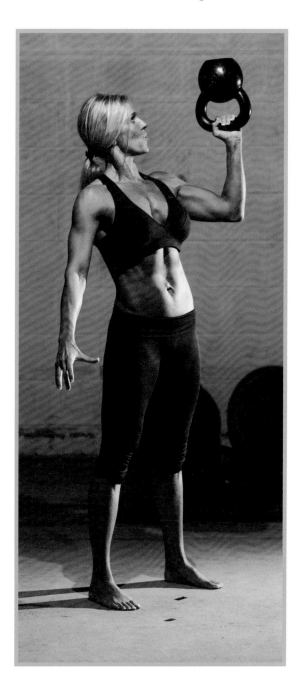
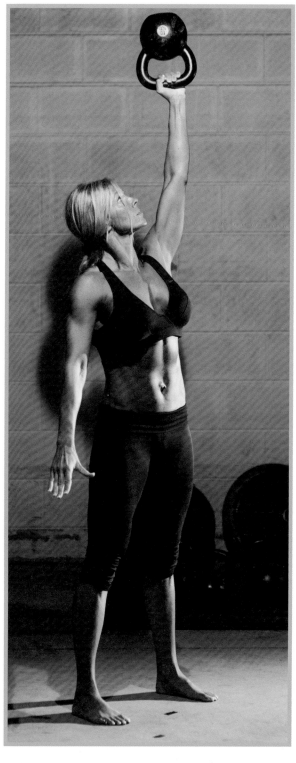

SEE-SAW PRESS

Begin with two bells in the rack position. Press one bell overhead. While lowering the first kettlebell back into the rack, simultaneously press the second kettlebell overhead. Continue alternating the presses.

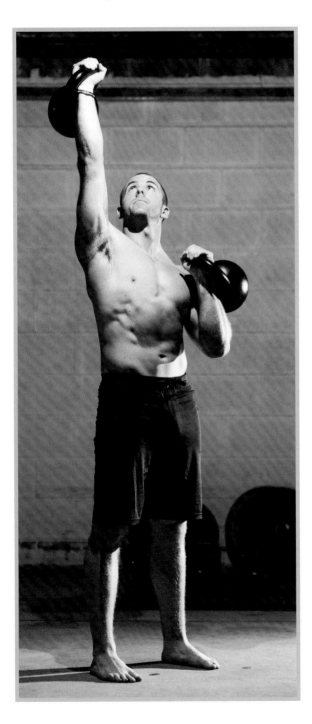 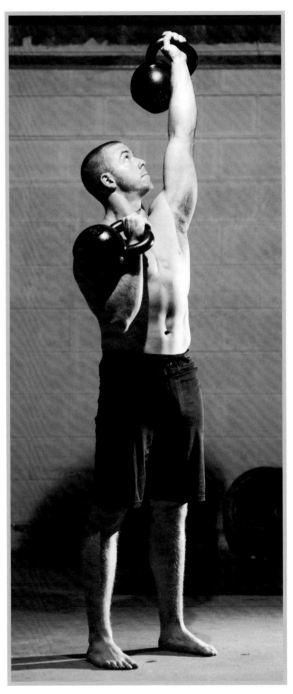

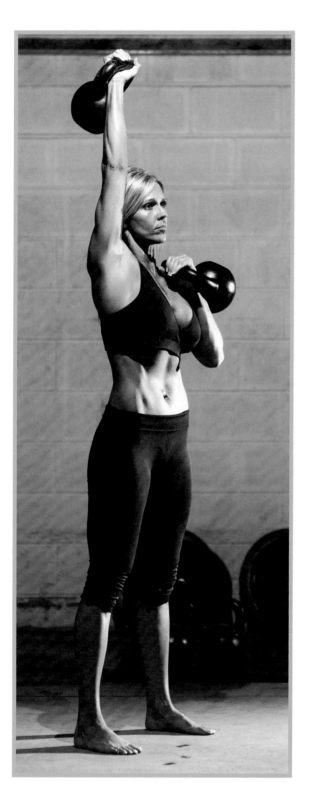
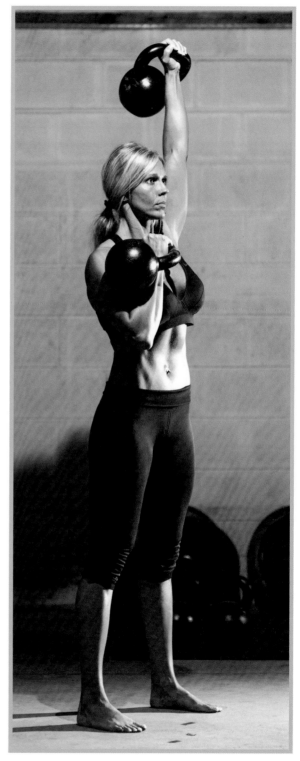

PALM PRESS

With your hand at the shoulder, start with the ball of one kettlebell in the palm of your hand. Make sure the handle faces away from you. Keep your eyes on the kettlebell and press it overhead.

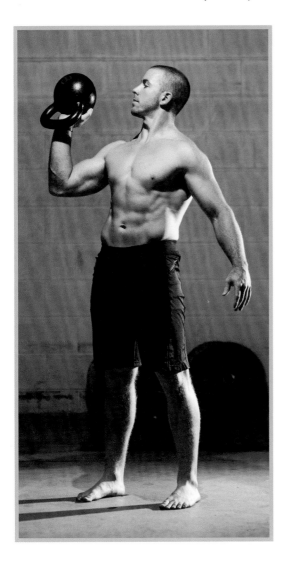
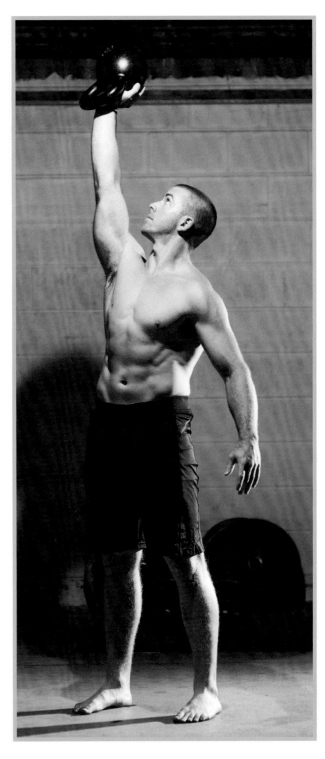

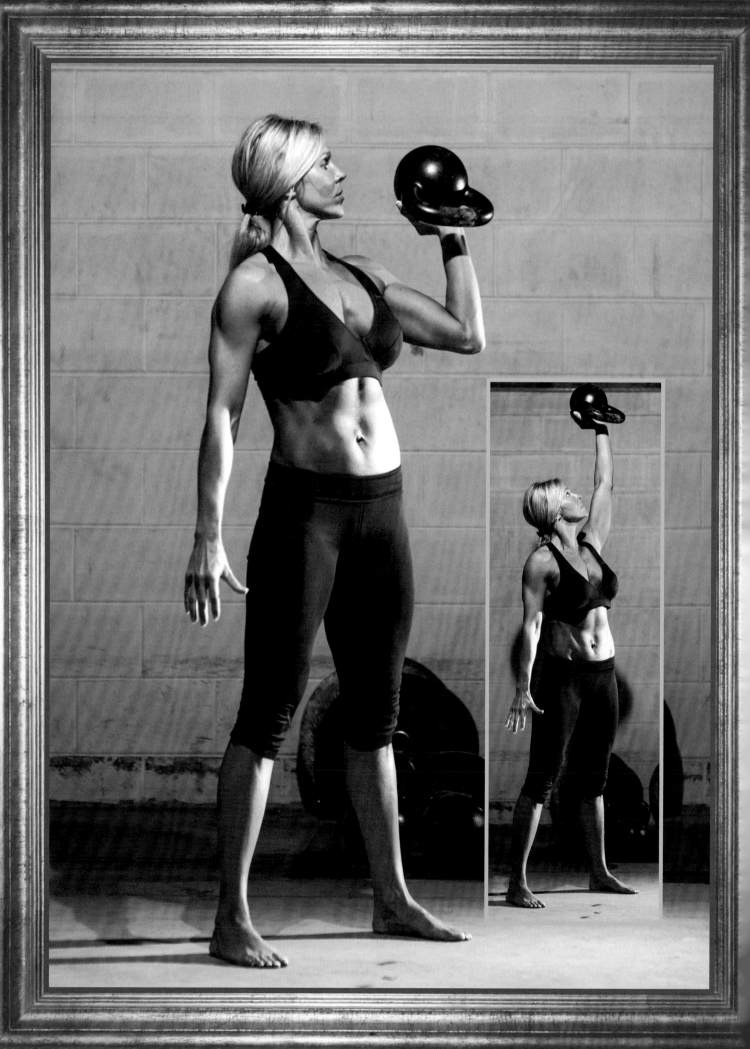

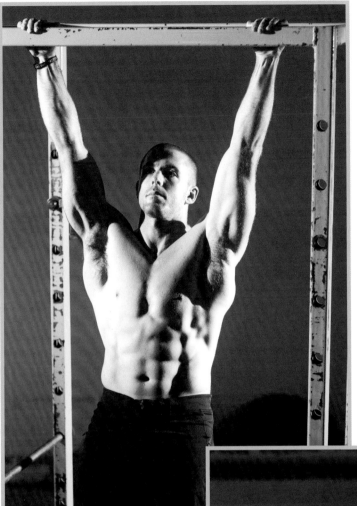

VERTICAL PULLING:

PULL-UP

Begin by hanging from a pull-up bar with a pronated (palms away) grip. Pull up until the bar is touching the sternum.

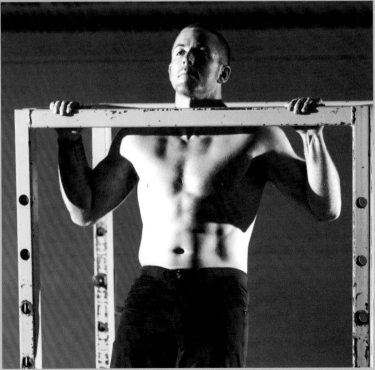

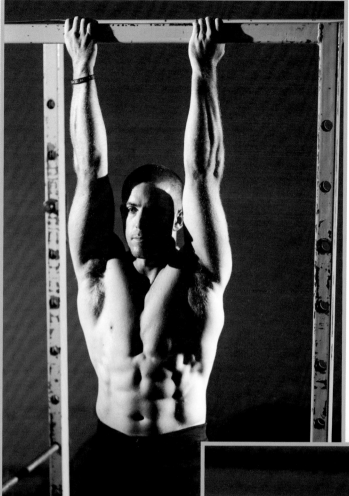

CHIN-UP

Hang from a pull-up bar with a supinated grip (palms facing toward you) Pull up until the bar is touching the sternum.

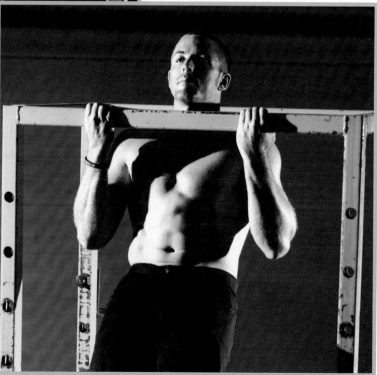

LAT PULLDOWN

Using a cable system, pull down until the bar touches the sternum. Can be done with a pronated or supinated grip as a remedial exercise for chin-ups and pull-ups.

HORIZONTAL PUSHING:
BILATERAL:

PUSH-UP

Assume a push-up position on the floor with hands underneath shoulders, arms straight, and feet together. Lower yourself down, keeping elbows in close to the body, until your chest (not your head) touches the floor. Press back up until arms are straight again, keeping the body supported.

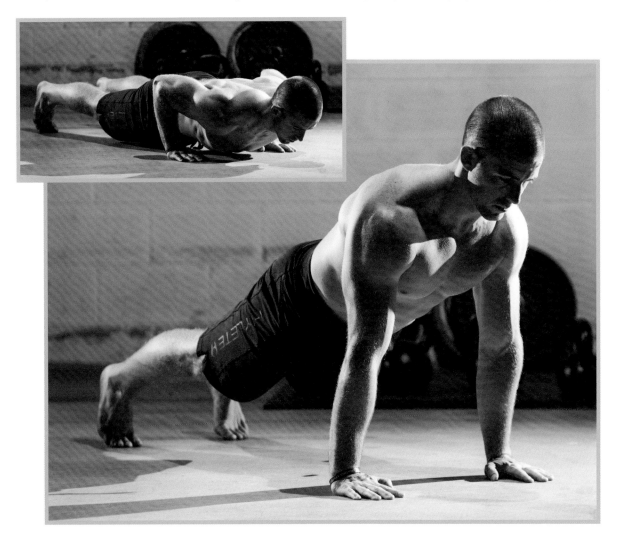

FLOOR PRESS

Lie supine on the floor with a pair of kettlebells held in the rack position. Press the bells to a full lockout, then lower them back down to the rack under control.

BENCH PRESS

Lie supine on a bench with a pair of kettlebells at the chest, press them to a full lockout, then lower them back down to the rack position under control

UNILATERAL:

ONE ARM FLOOR PRESS

Lie supine on the floor with a kettlebell held in the rack position. Press it to a full lockout, then lower it back down to the rack under control.

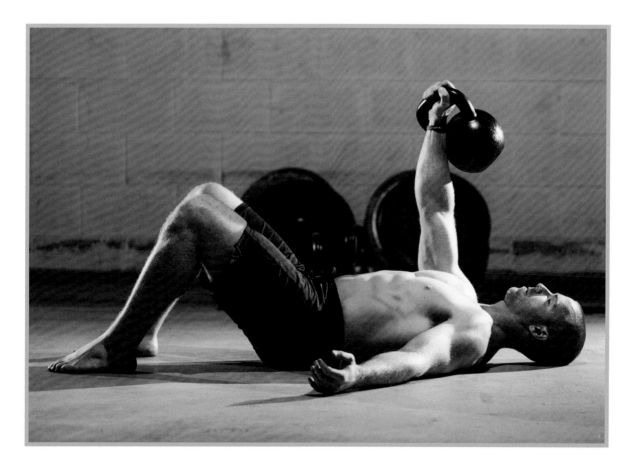

ONE ARM BENCH PRESS

Lie supine on a bench with a kettlebell in the rack position. Press it to a full lockout, then lower it under control.

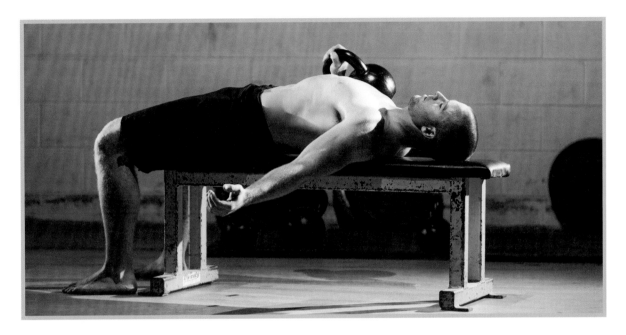

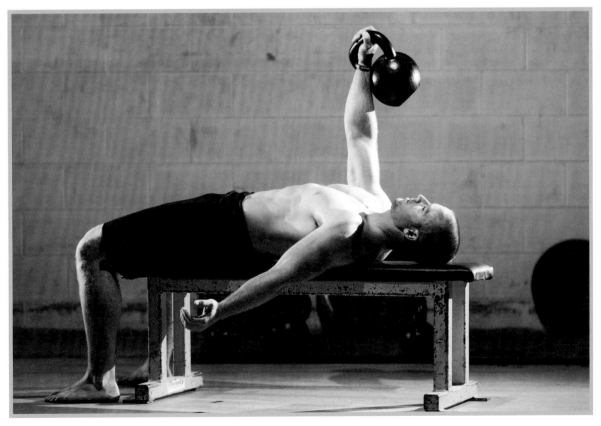

HORIZONTAL PULLING:
BILATERAL:

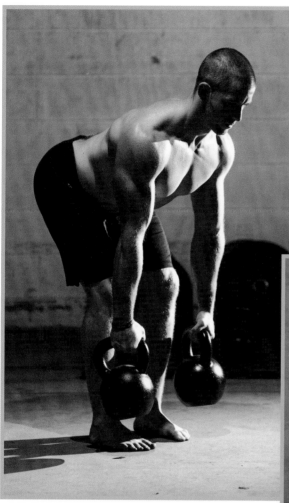

BENT OVER ROW

Stand with a kettlebell in each hand. Keep a straight back and bend over by reaching the hips back. Maintaining this position, row the kettlebells to the chest then slowly lower them back to the start position under control.

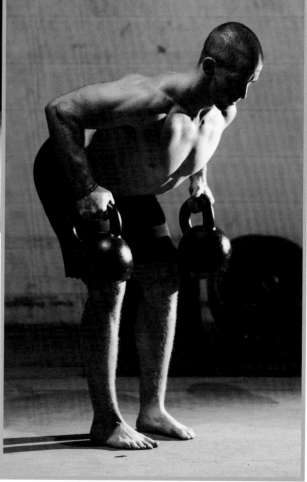

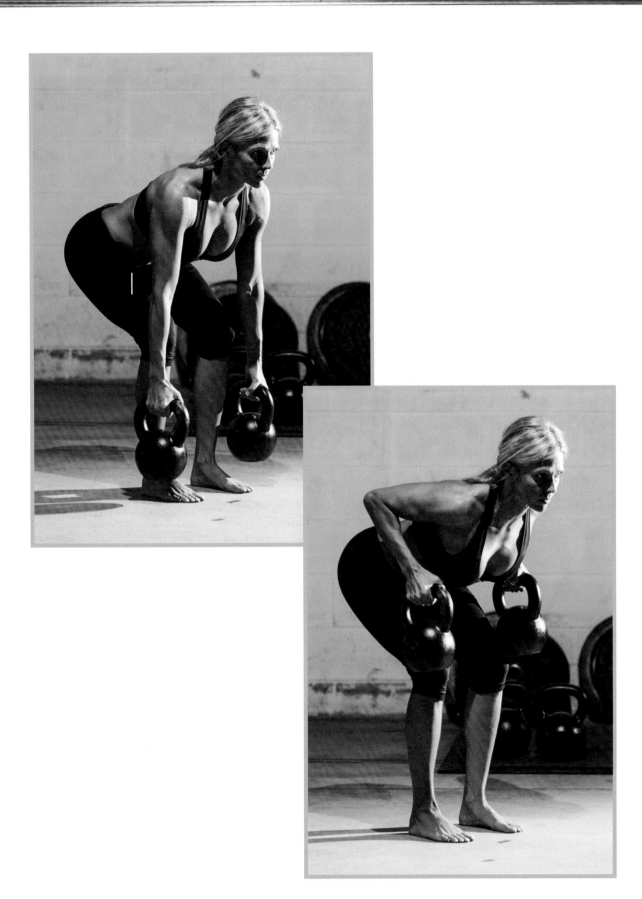

UNILATERAL:

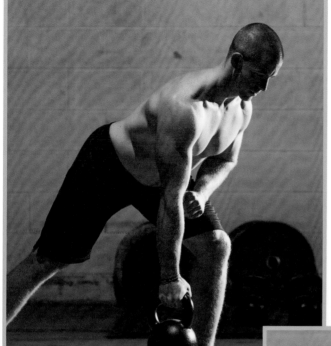

ONE ARM SUPPORTED ROW

While holding one kettlebell, reach the opposite leg forward and place the forearm of this same side on the thigh for support. For example, if holding the kettlebell in the right hand, the left leg would be forward with the left forearm on the thigh. From this position, row the kettlebell to the chest while maintaining good posture.

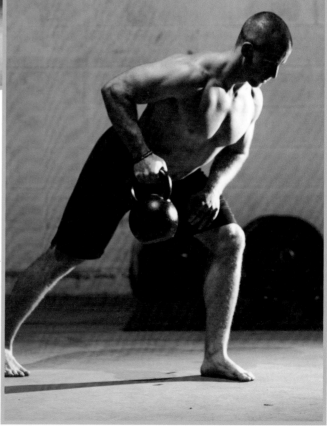

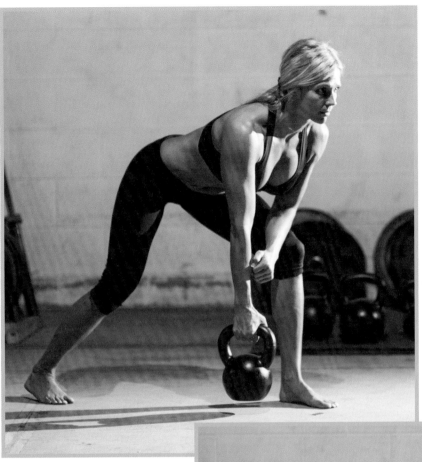

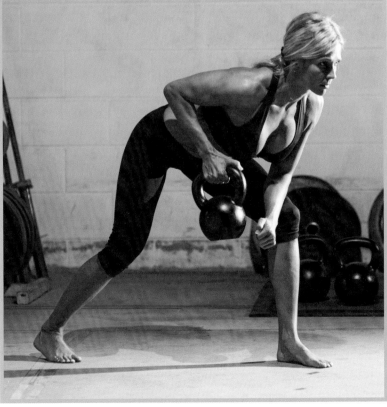

ONE ARM UNSUPPORTED ROW

While holding one kettlebell, assume an asymmetrical stance, with the opposite leg forward. Row the kettlebell to the chest without using the free arm for support. Emphasize good posture through core strength. The front leg, especially the glute will have to work harder in order to stabilize during this movement.

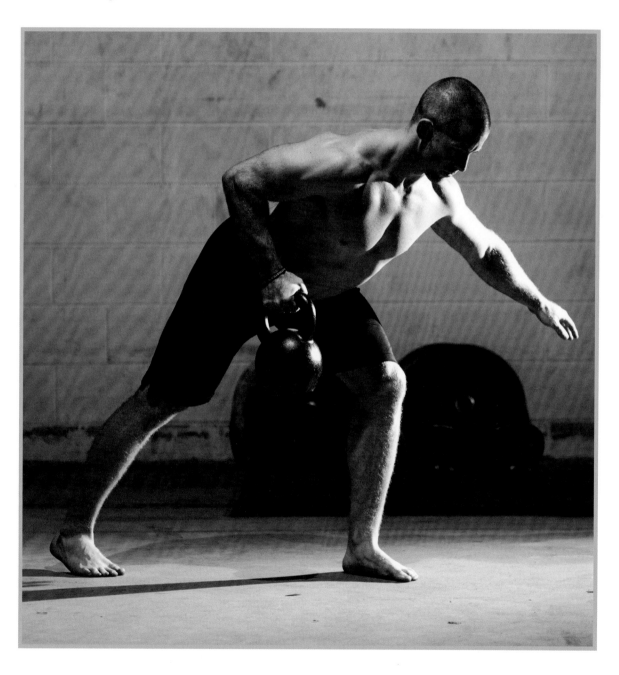

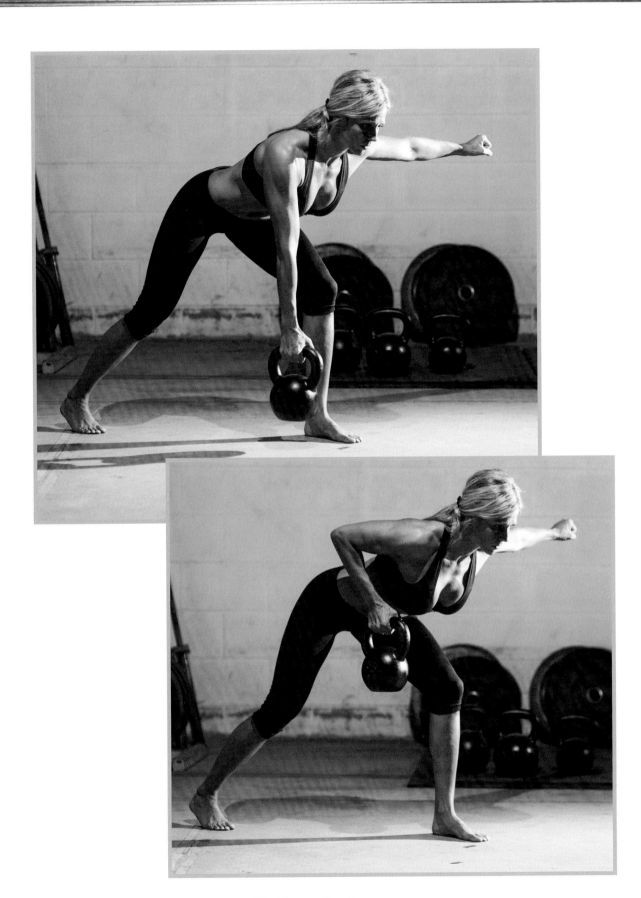

RENEGADE ROW

From a push-up position with wide feet, grip a pair of kettlebells. Maintain a neutral spine and perform alternating rows.

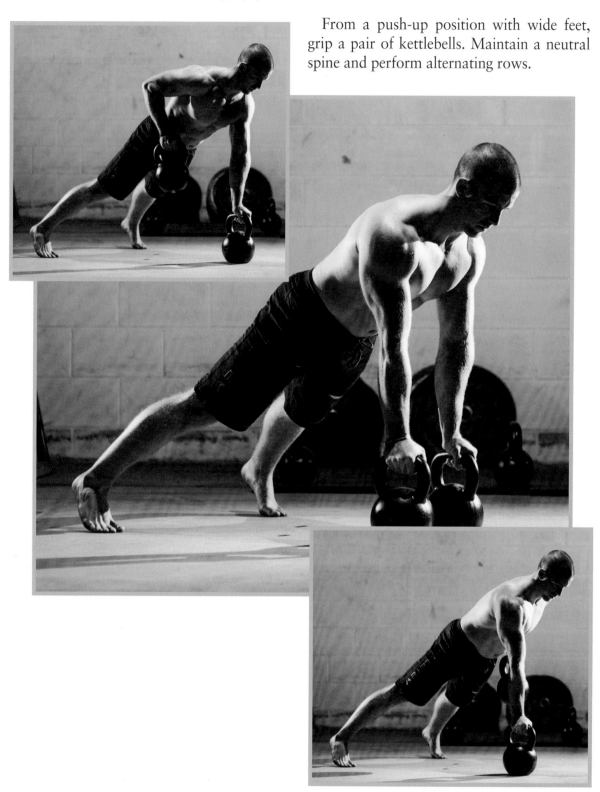

LOWER BODY:
KNEE DOMINANT (PUSH):
BILATERAL:

SQUAT

Assume a comfortable shoulder-width stance with feet slightly turned out. Descend into a squat while maintaining a good spinal curve and keeping the heels down. Squeeze the glutes to stand up. (See the Exercises section for an in-depth description of the squat.)

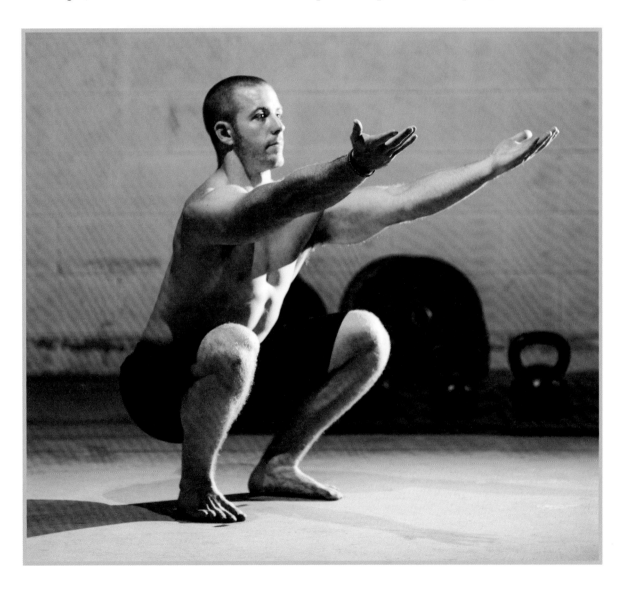

GOBLET SQUAT

Using a comfortable shoulder width stance, hold a kettlebell by the handles ("horns") with both hands at the chest. Sit back into a squat and use your elbows on the inside of the knees to enhance flexibility of the hips while maintaining good posture. Return to standing.

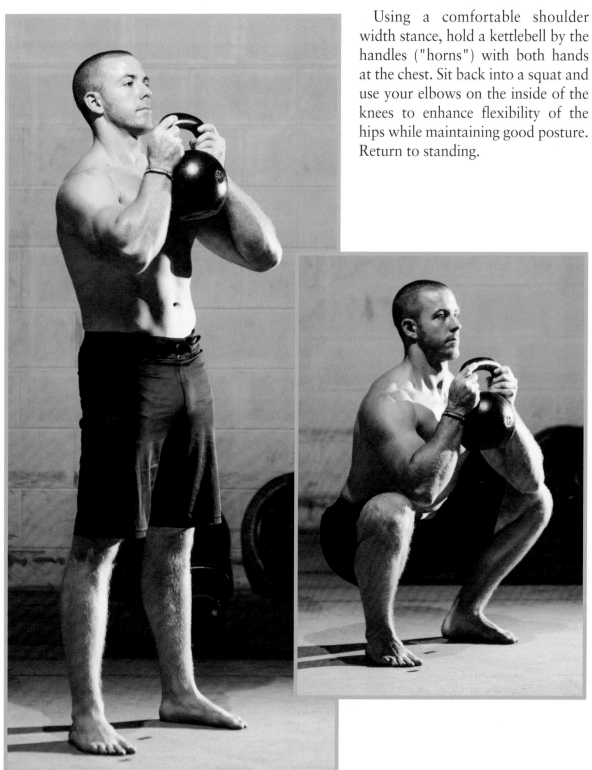

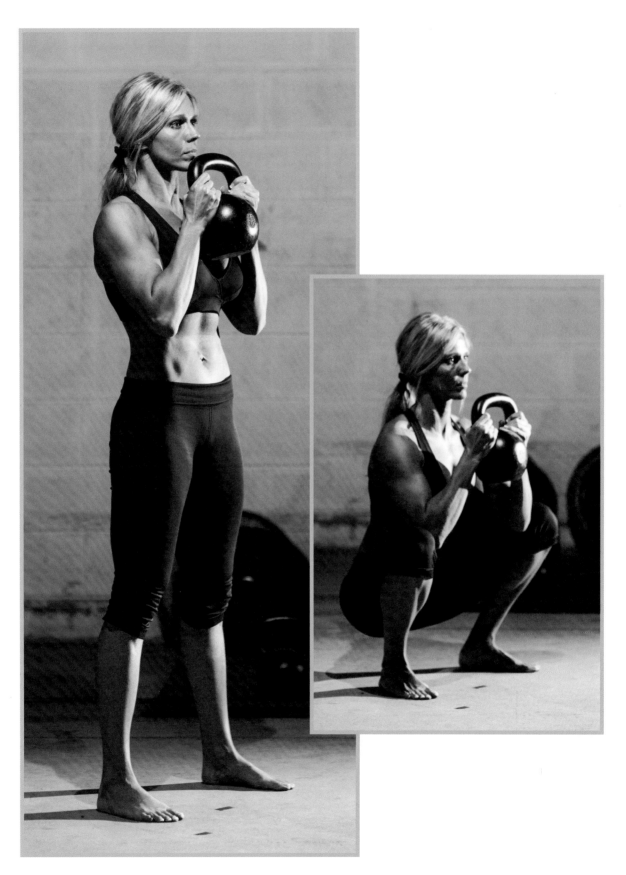

FRONT SQUAT

Bring one or two kettlebells to the rack position, descend into a squat and return to standing.

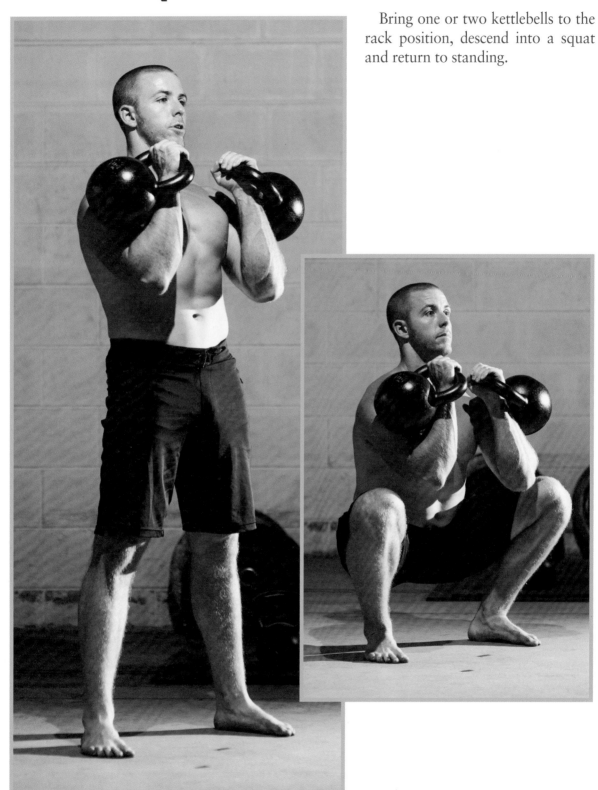

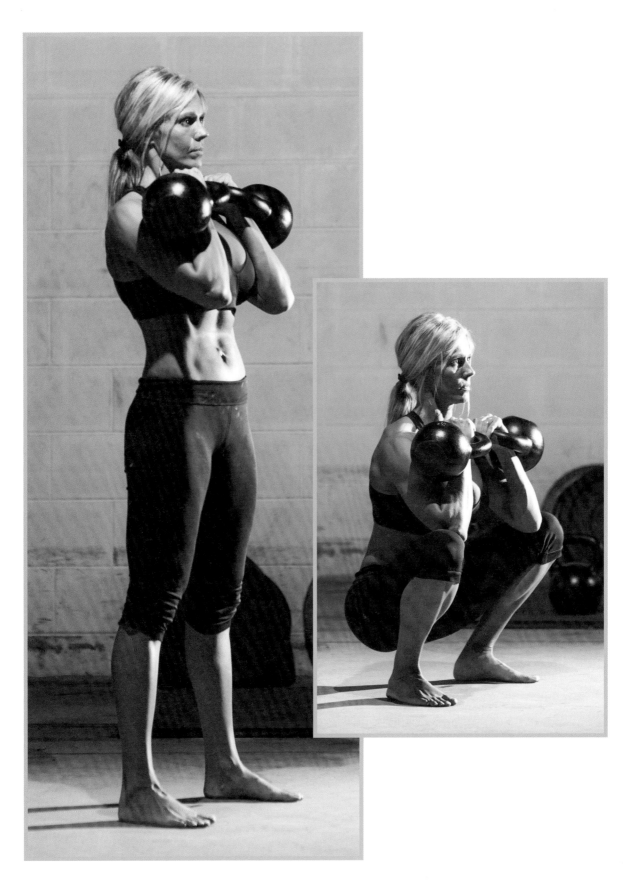

OVERHEAD SQUAT

Press one or two kettlebells overhead. Perform squats while keeping the kettlebell(s) overhead.

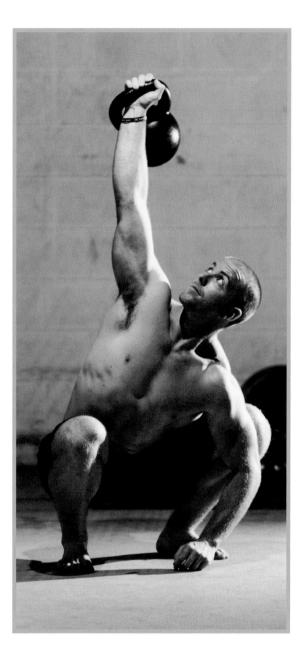
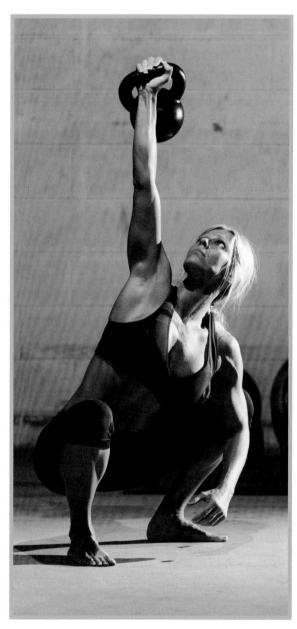

UNILATERAL:

SPLIT SQUAT

Assume an asymmetrical stance with one leg forward. Descend until the rear knee softly touches the floor. Drive through the front heel to return to the asymmetrical stance. (See pictures for alternate kettlebell loading positions)

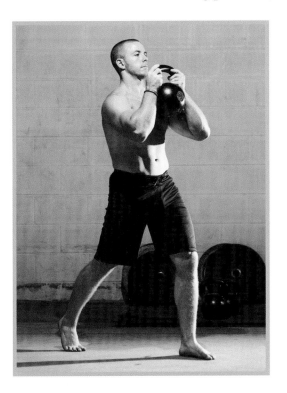
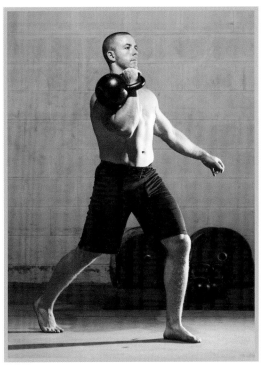
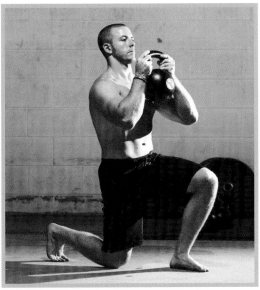
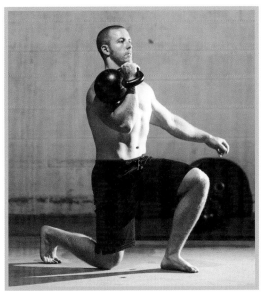

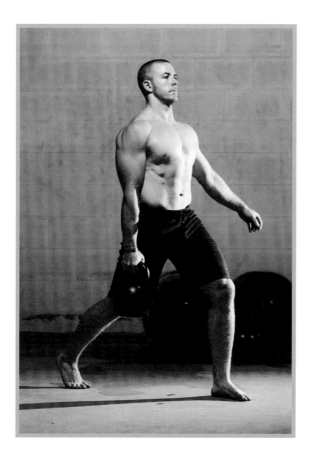
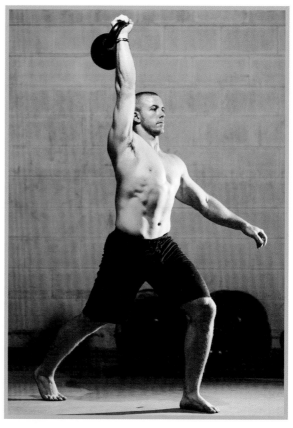
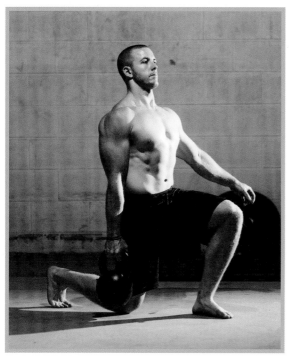
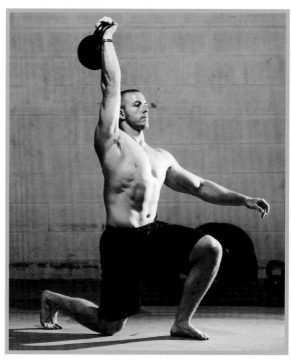

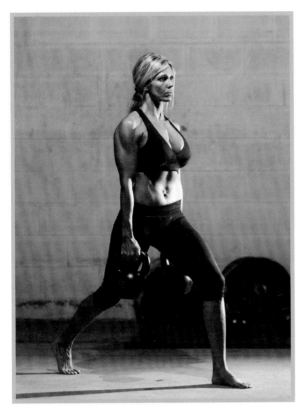
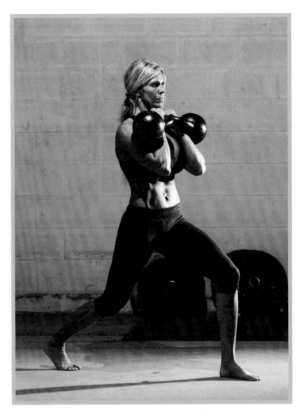
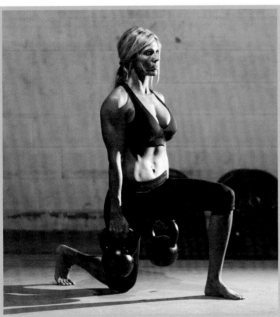
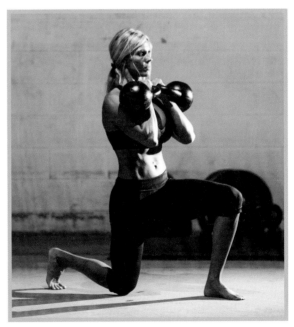

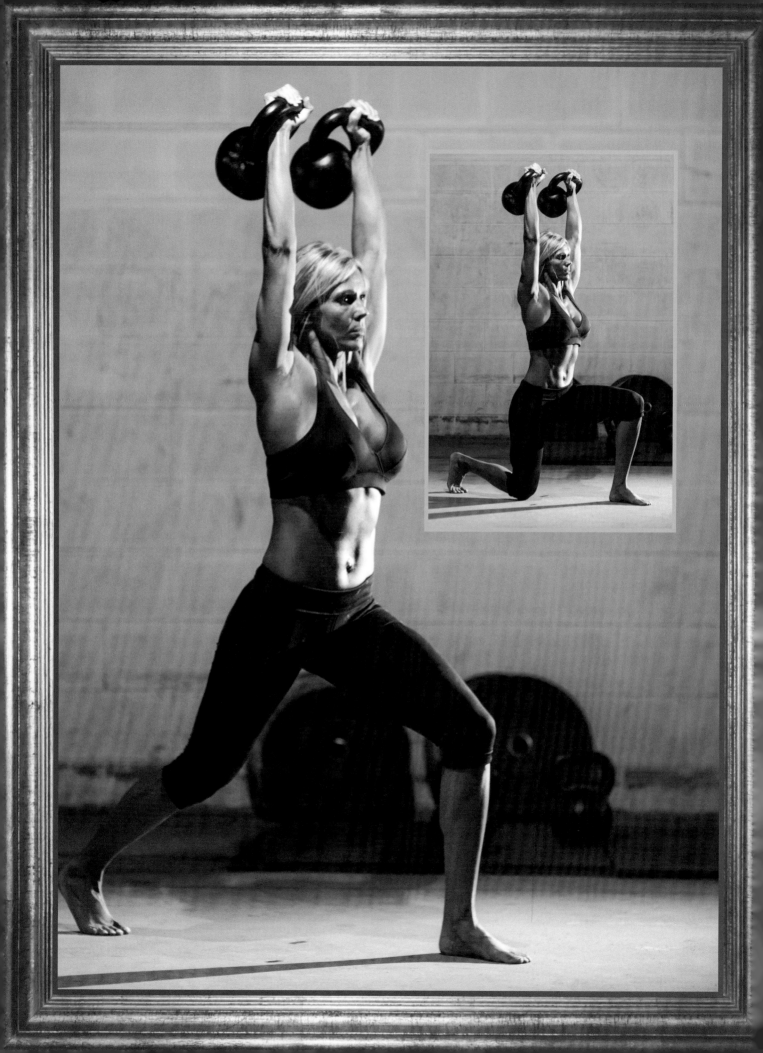

FORWARD LUNGE

From a standing position, step forward into a lunge so that the rear knee softly touches the floor. Drive through the front heel to return to standing with feet together. (See pictures for alternate kettlebell loading positions)

REVERSE LUNGE

From a standing position, step backward into a lunge so that the rear knee touches the floor. Drive through the front heel to return to original standing position. (See pictures for alternate kettlebell loading positions)

AIRBORNE LUNGE

From a single leg standing position, reach the free knee to the floor without touching the free foot. Keeping the front heel down, return to standing.

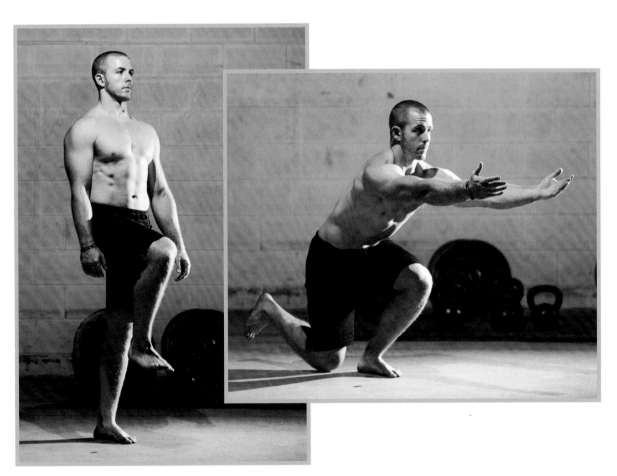

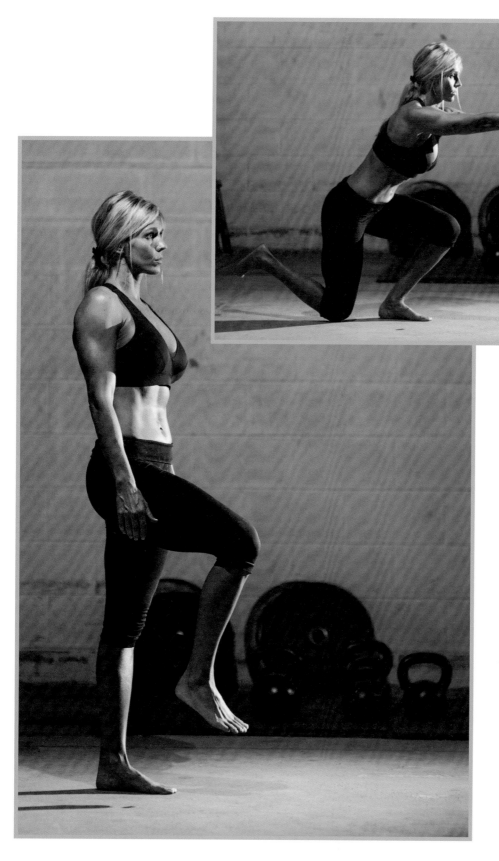

SINGLE LEG SQUAT

While standing on one leg, keep the your heel down while descending into a squat of an appropriate depth. Push through the heel to return to standing. It is best to start this movement by sitting back to a high box to control the range of motion at first until you can safely and gradually work your way down to full range of motion.

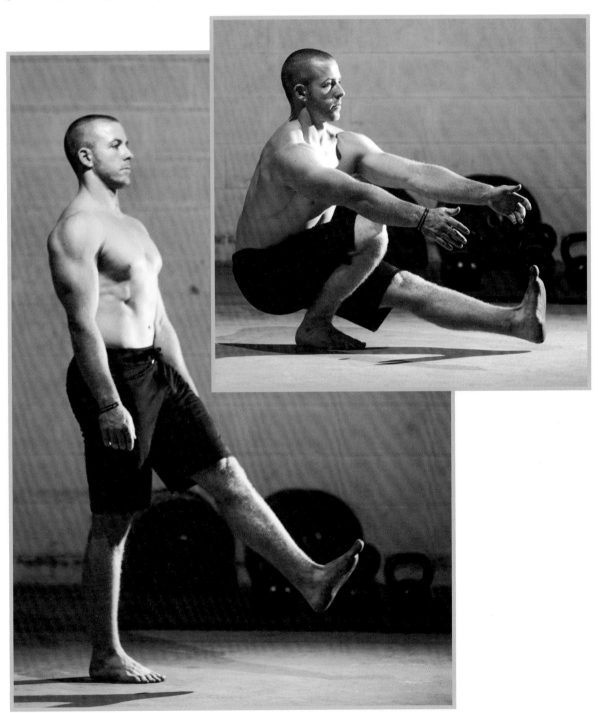

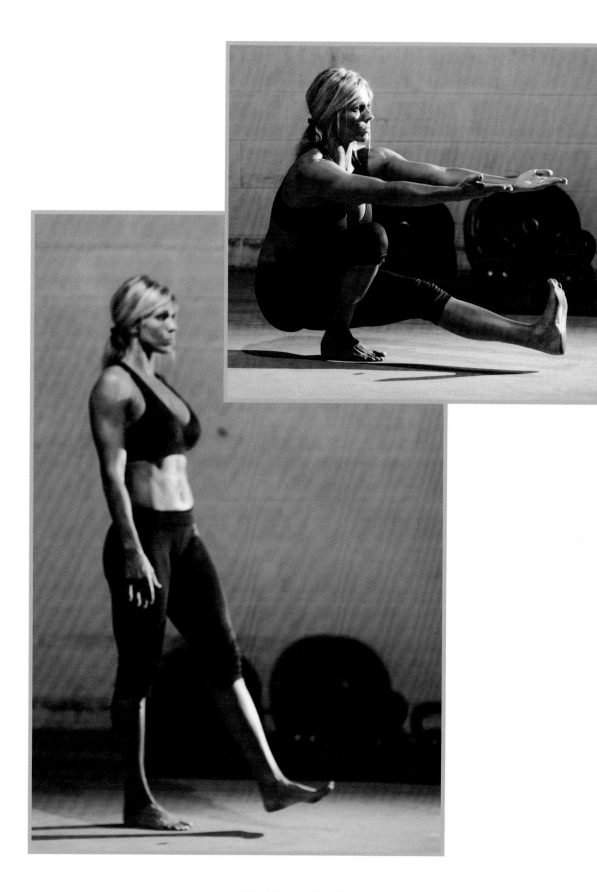

HIP DOMINANT (PULL):
BILATERAL:

DEADLIFT

Start in a standing position with kettlebell held in both hands. Perform deadlifts.

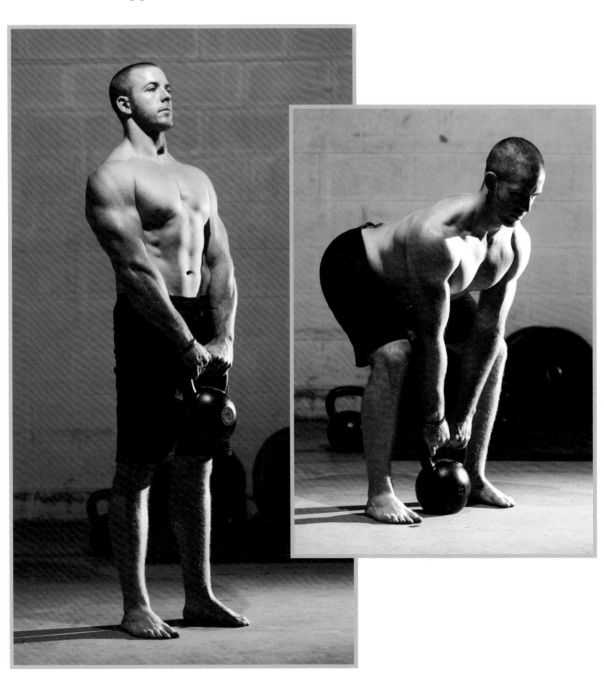

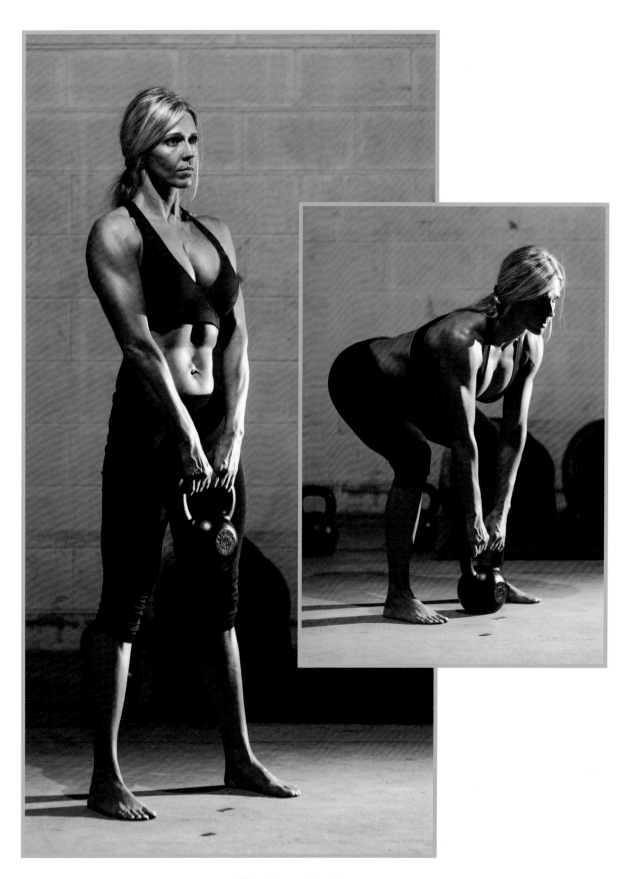

SUMO DEADLIFT

Assume a wider than normal deadlift stance and perform the standard deadlift with one or two kettlebells. This stance will be necessary for using double weights.

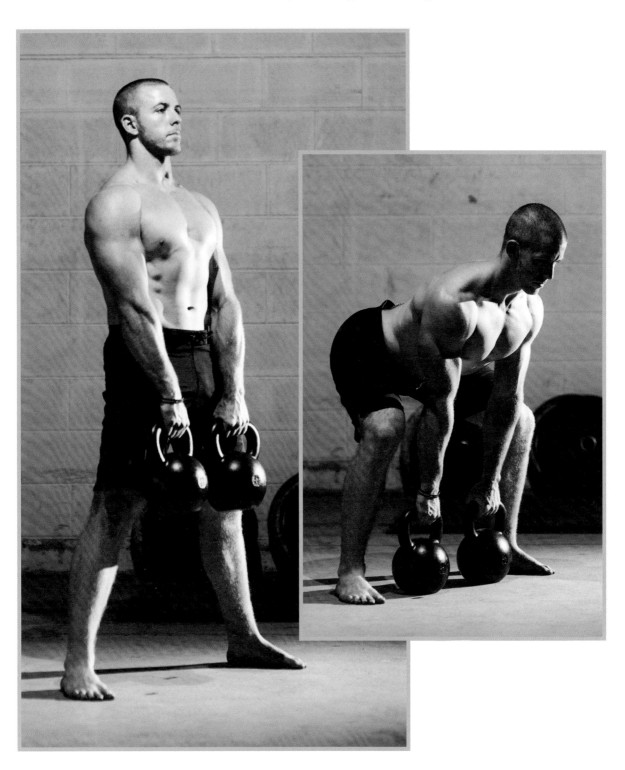

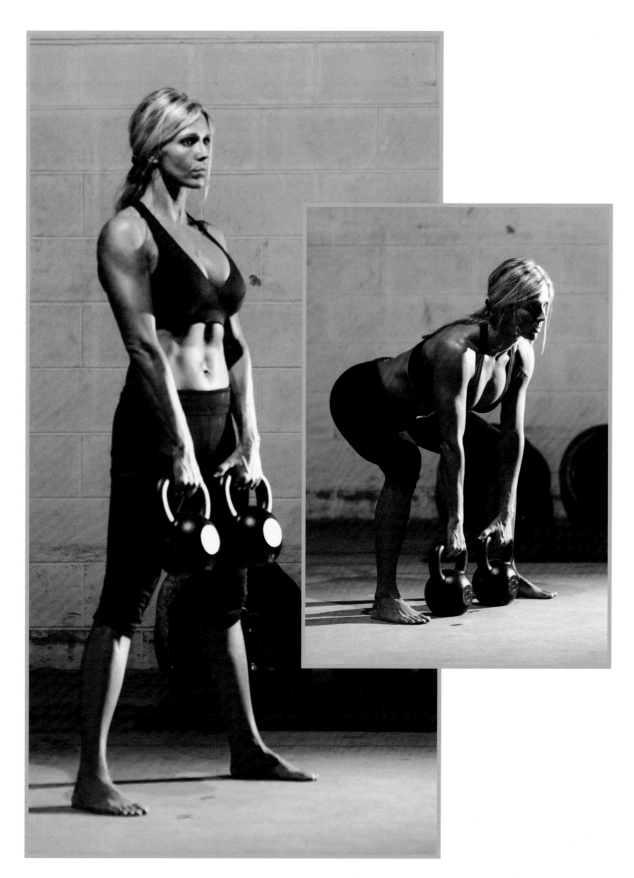

ROMANIAN DEADLIFT

With minimal knee bend, perform deadlifts with one or two kettlebells.

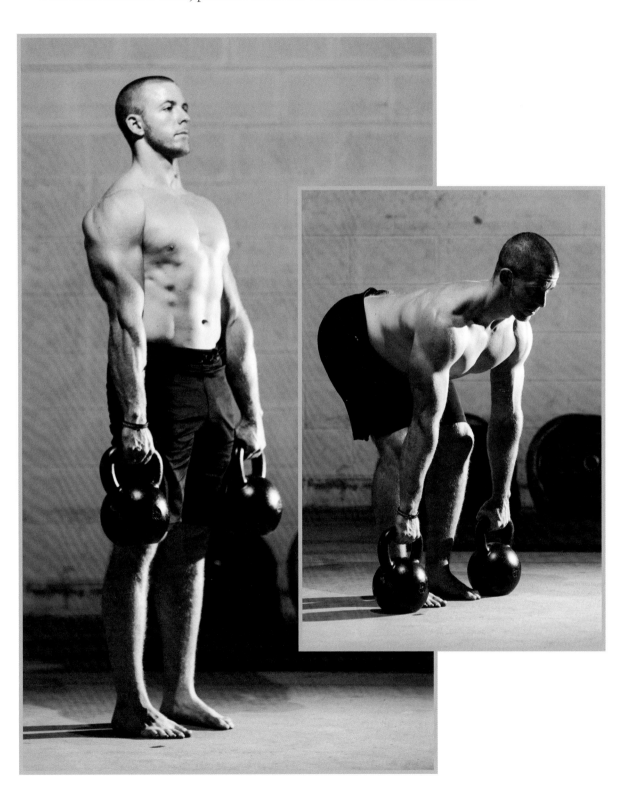

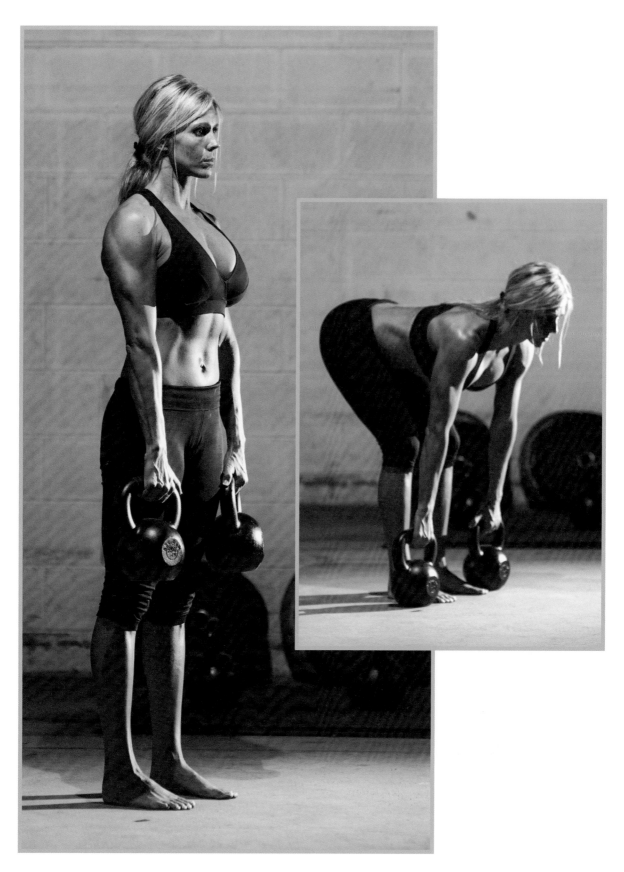

GLUTE BRIDGE

Lie supine on the floor with heels down. Drive the hips upward using the glutes.

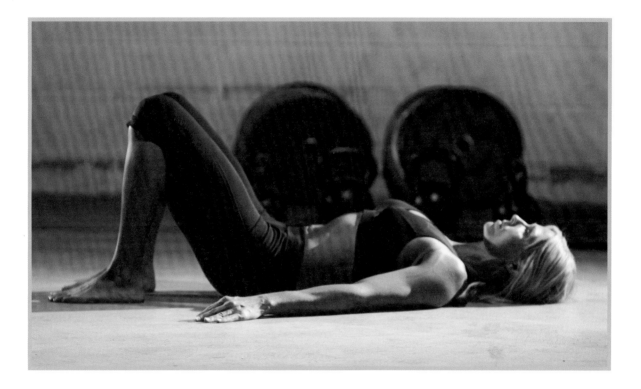

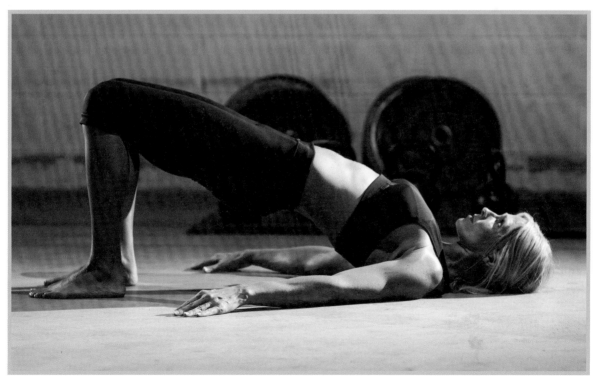

SWING

See full description in Exercises.

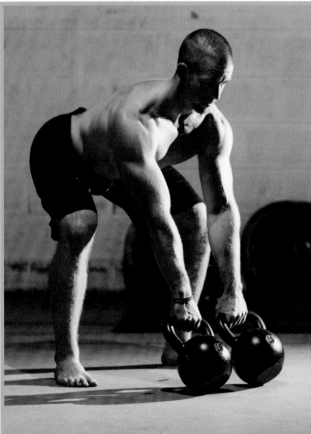

DOUBLE SWING

Perform swings with two kettlebells.

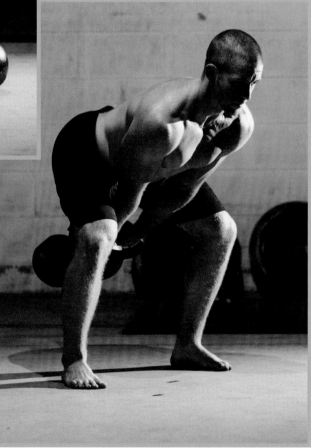

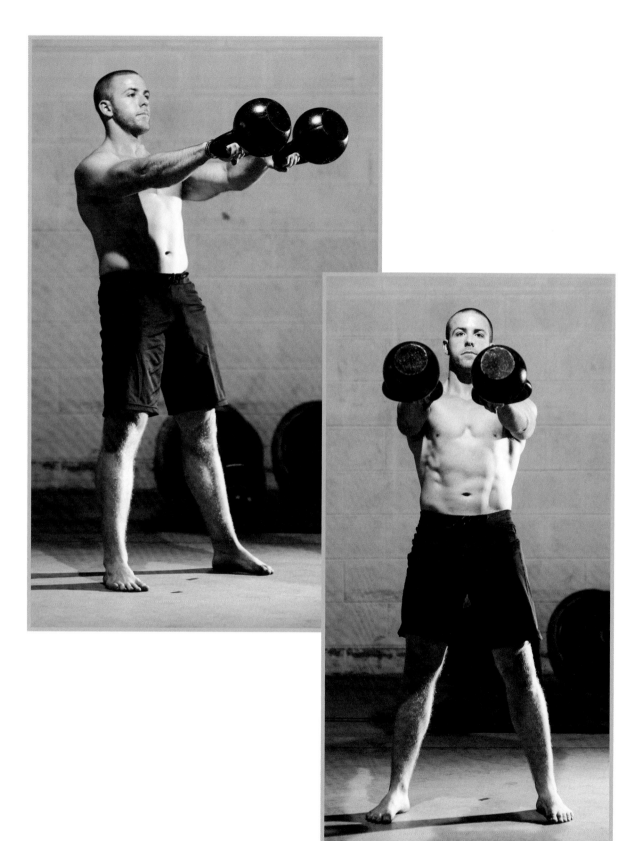

SNATCH

See full description in Exercises.

DOUBLE SNATCH

Perform snatches with two kettlebells. Pull the kettlebells down to the rack position before snatching again.

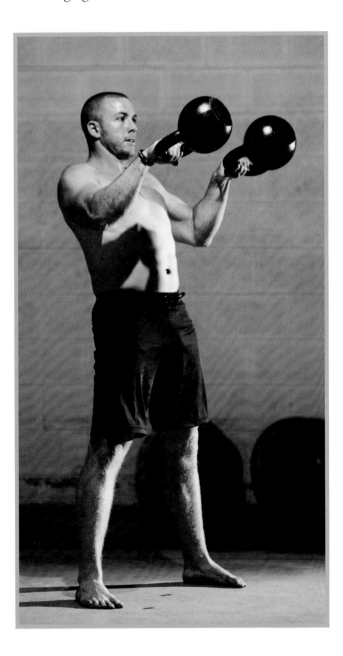
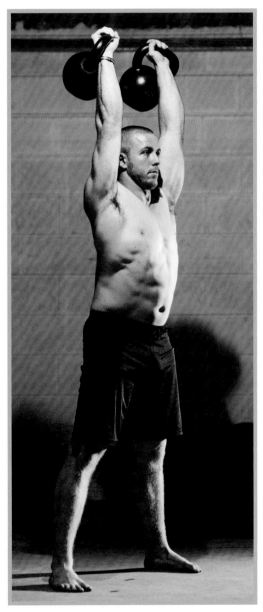

CLEAN

See full description in Exercises.

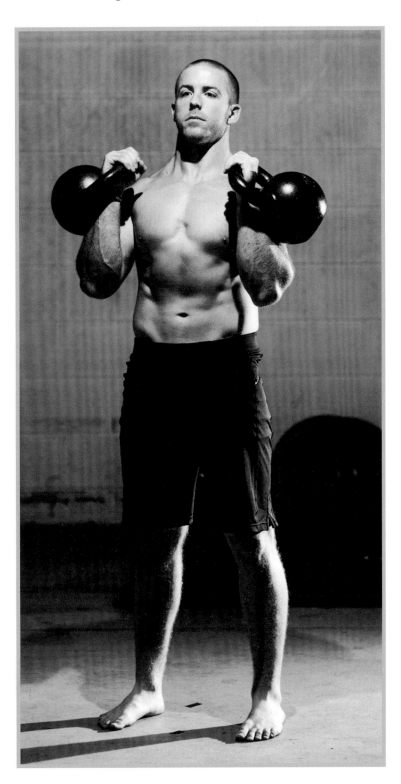

DOUBLE CLEAN

Perform cleans with two kettlebells, take care not to let the kettlebells bang together at the top to protect the fingers.

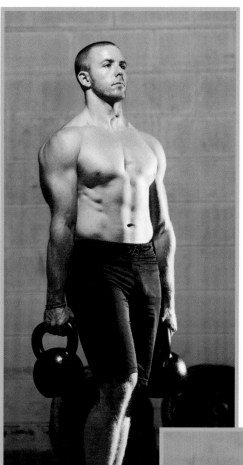

UNILATERAL:

SINGLE LEG DEADLIFT

Holding a kettlebell in one or both hands, stand on one leg and perform deadlifts. Lift the free leg up and back while maintaining good posture during the descent.

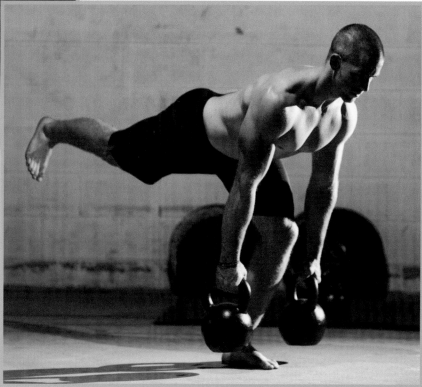

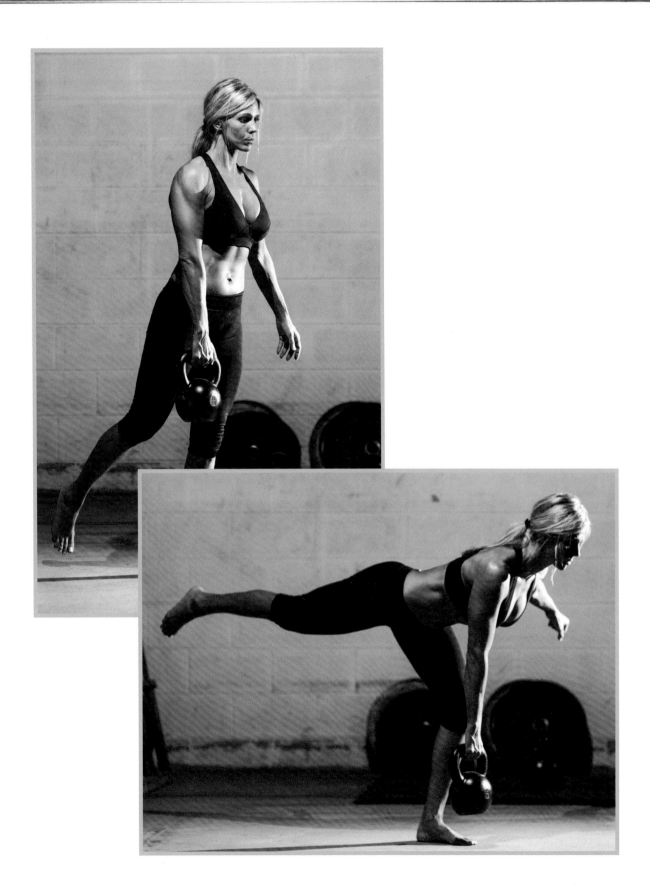

SINGLE LEG BRIDGE

Perform bridges using only one leg. Hold the free leg close to the chest.

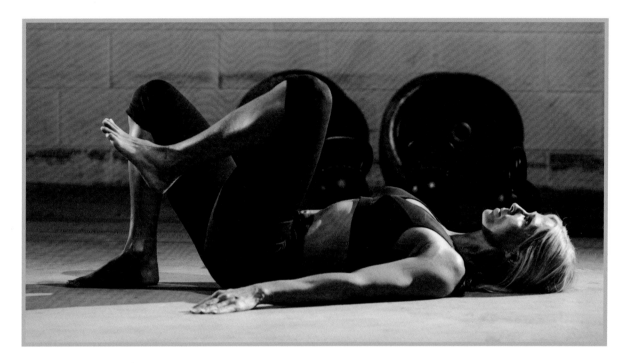

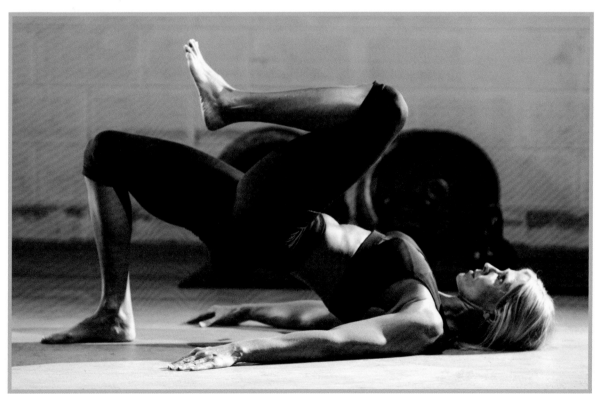

CORE EXERCISES:

STABILITY:

Please note the absence of crunches, sit-ups, and other traditional forward bending abdominal exercises. Not only does excessive forward bending reinforce poor posture, it also has been scientifically shown (Stu McGill) to deteriorate the intervertebral discs.

PLANK

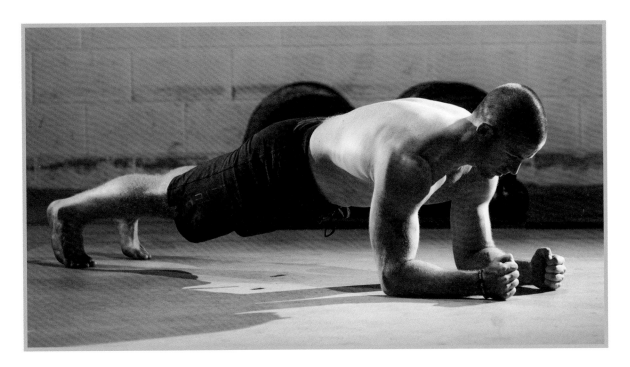

SHOULDER TAPS

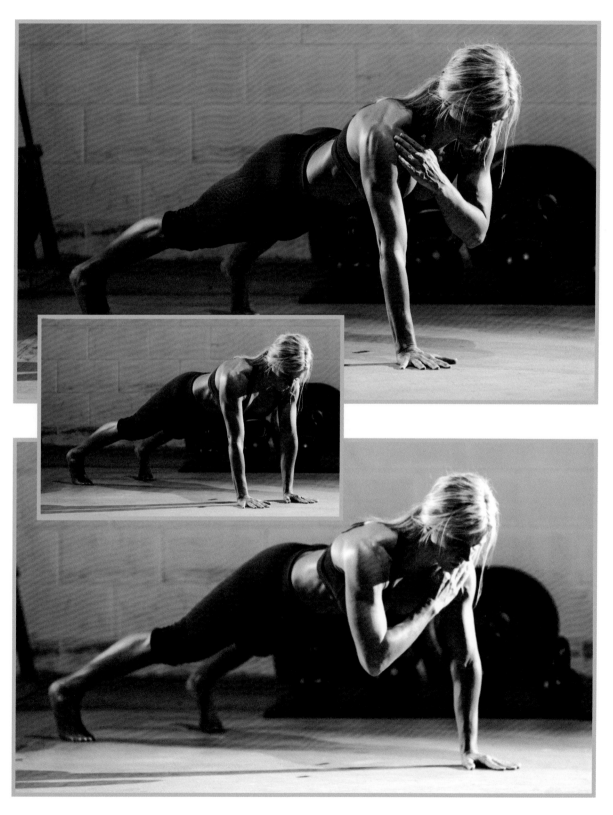

ONE ARM PLANK

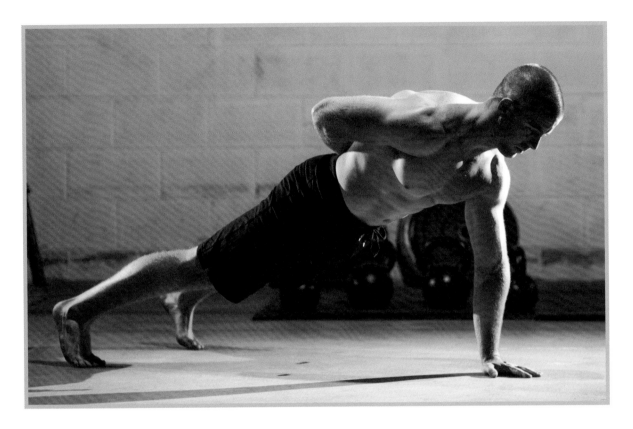

RENEGADE ROW

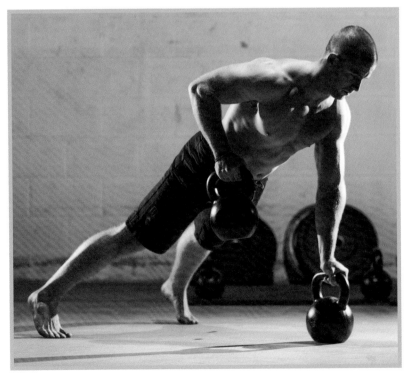

ACTIVE LEG LOWERING

Bring both legs to vertical from laying down. Keep one leg as high as possible while lowering the other leg under control until the calf touches the floor. Return to start position and repeat on both sides.

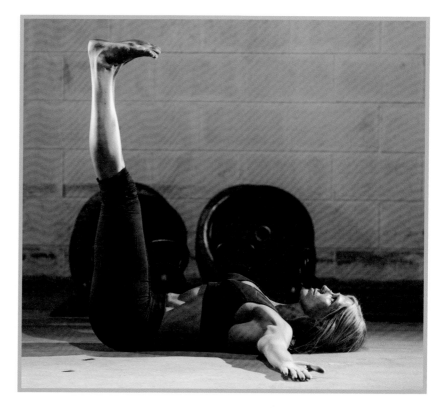

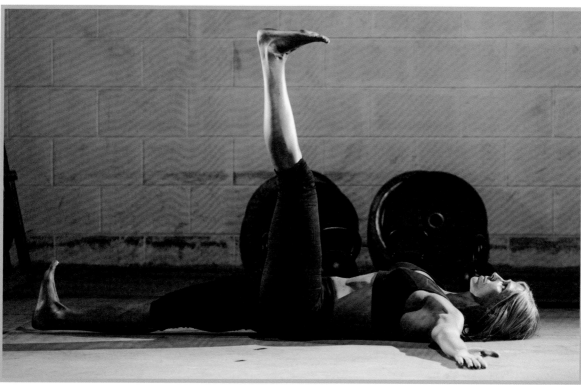

SIDE PLANK

Side Planks are a great exercise to ensure stability through the pelvis and trunk. It specifically targets muscle groups that are meant to stabilize the pelvis and core which will help alleviate many common movement impairments.

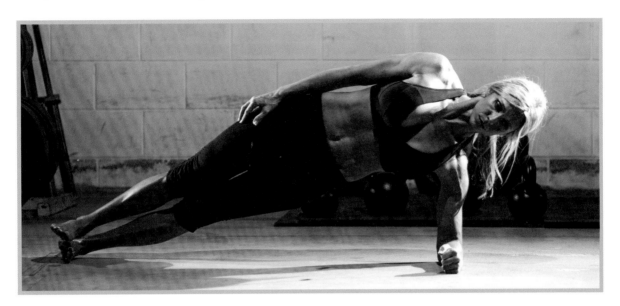

ADVANCED SIDE PLANK

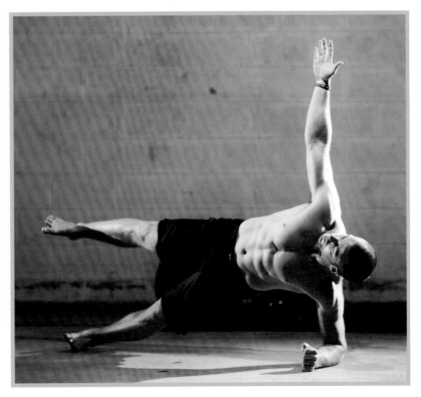

ONE ARM CARRIES

Loaded carries are great for working the core and for developing proper core-firing patterns. Use as a finisher, a core exercise, or a warm-up.

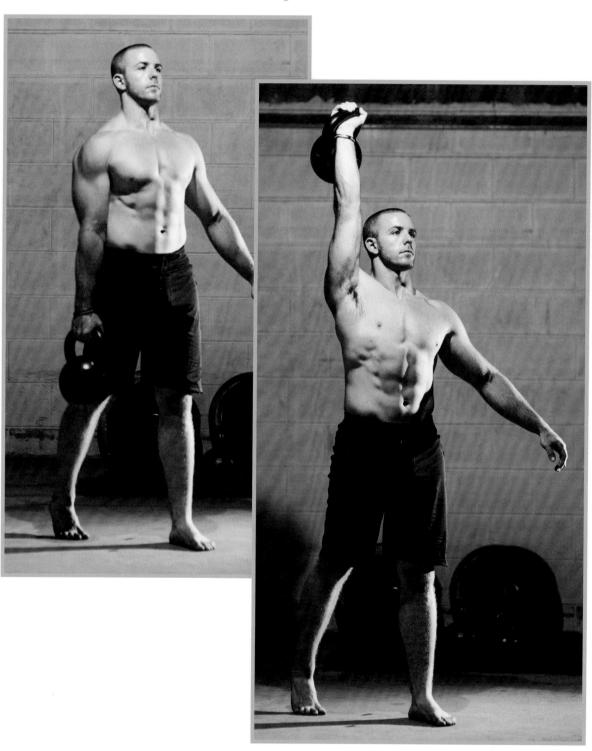

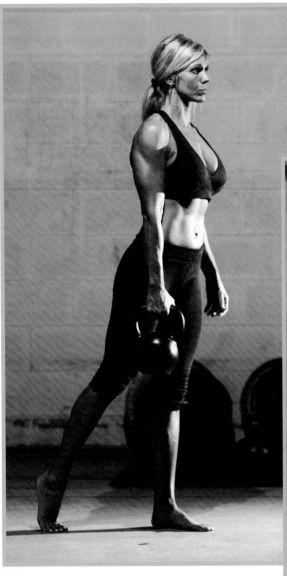

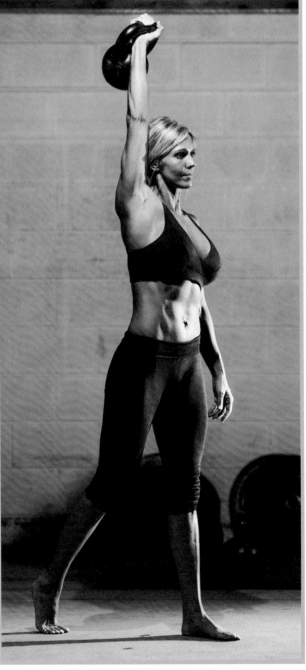

"WHAT IF I WANT TO WORK THE BICEPS?"

Even though the exercises in this book primarily focus on movements not individual muscles, the reason many people come to you as a trainer is to look better, or look more fit. In some situations, isolation exercises can be beneficial for stimulating a specific body part. The following exercises have a decent bang for your buck for aesthetics as well as improving grip and core strength. Use these exercises at the end of the exercise session as the "icing on the cake" while keeping the primary focus of your training on larger movements such as presses, pushups, rows, pull-ups, and squats.

ISOLATION EXERCISES:
SHOULDERS:

FRONT RAISE

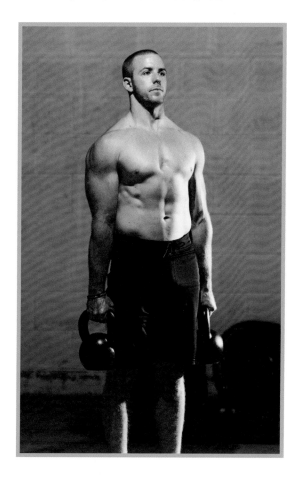
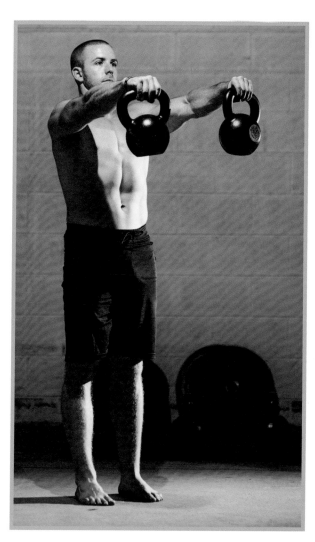

SIDE RAISE

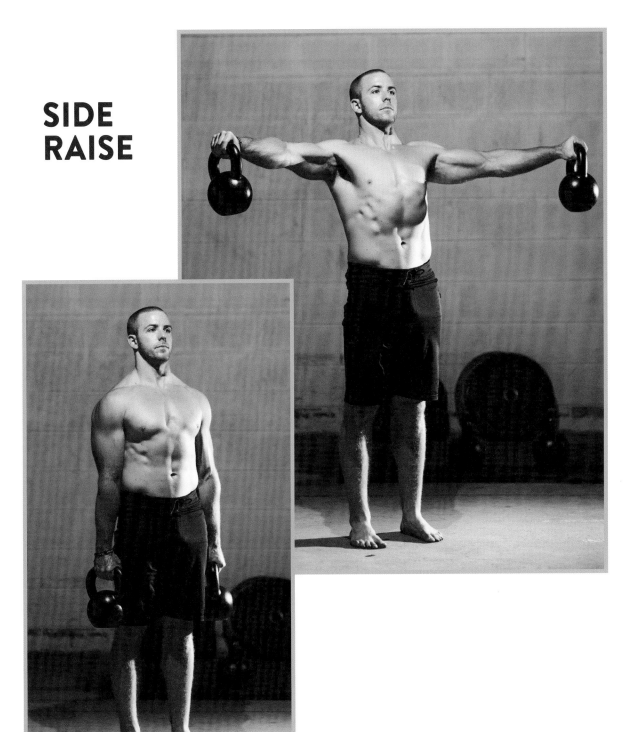

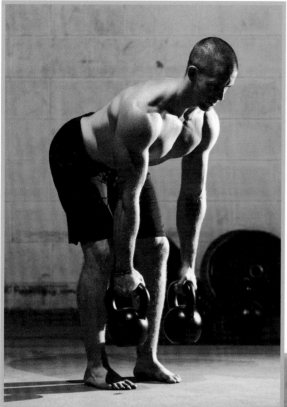

BACK:

REAR DELTOID FLY

This exercise should be performed with the same good bottom position of a dead-lift posture. This drill is great for improving middle and upper back strength and posture. Make sure to keep the shoulders away from the ears during this movement.

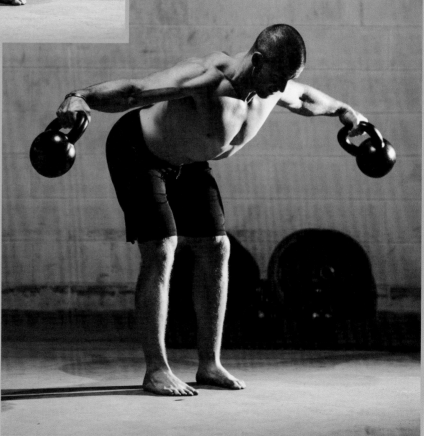

BICEPS:

CURL

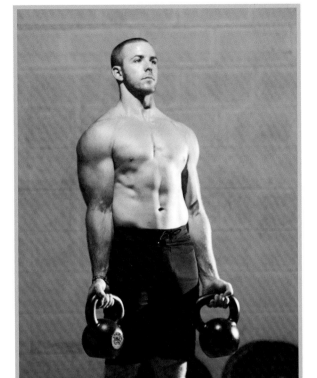

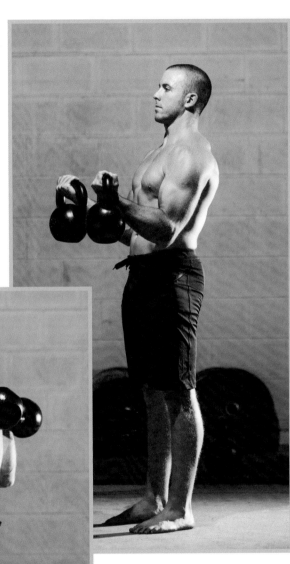

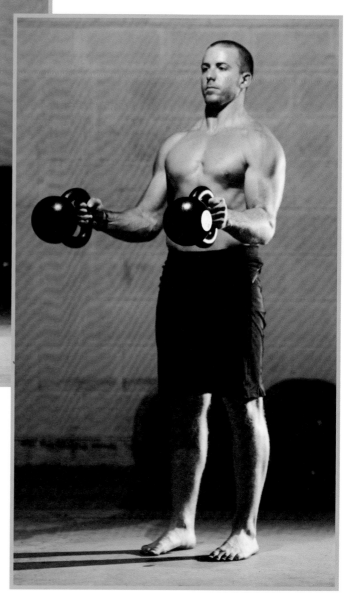

PITCHER CURL

The pitcher curl is not only a biceps exercise, but will target the grip, wrists, and forearms in a way that is hard to replicate. Wrist and grip strength will definitely be the limiting factor here, drill the pitcher curl for a vice grip and steel wrists.

TRICEPS:

PULLOVER

This drill is not only great for the triceps, but if performed correctly can also greatly improve shoulder mobility. Make sure to keep the shoulders down away from the ears on this drill and go only as far as your flexibility will allow.

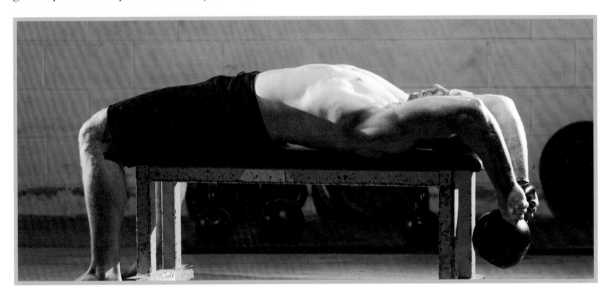

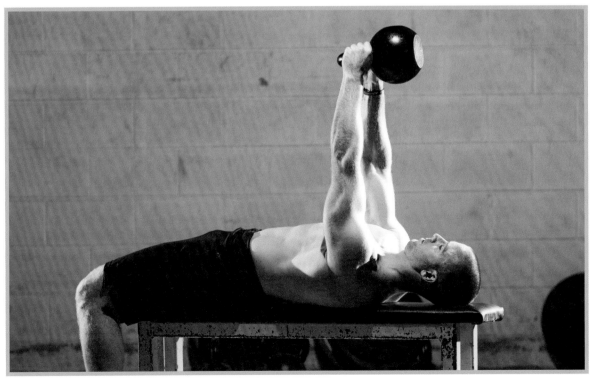

FRENCH PRESS

CLOSE GRIP PUSH-UP

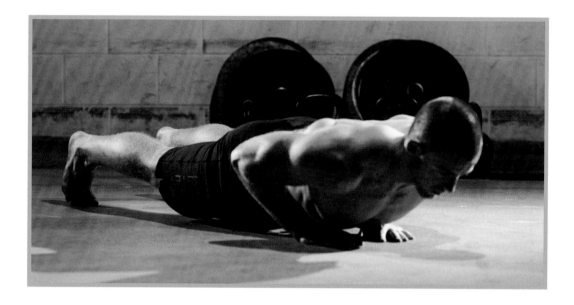

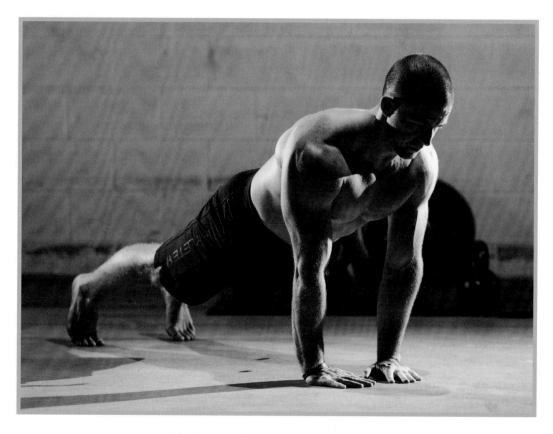

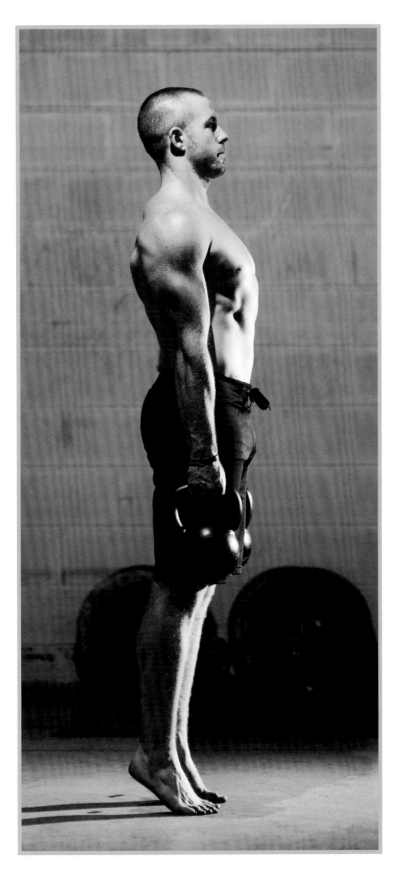

CALVES:

CALF RAISE WITH KETTLEBELL

These isolation exercises should only be supplemental, and not the focus of a balanced program. The main exercise movements will already target all of these muscle groups synergistically.

- Upper body pulling will generally use the lats, traps, rear deltoids, biceps, and forearms.
- Upper body pushing will use the shoulders, pecs, and triceps.
- Lower body pushing will use the entire musculature of the leg emphasizing the quadriceps.
- Lower body pulling will use the entire musculature of the leg emphasizing the glutes and hamstrings.

PUTTING IT ALL TOGETHER
TEMPLATE:

Superset
> Upper Body Push + Lower Body Pull

Superset
> Upper Body Pull + Lower Body Push

Isolation and Core Exercises

SAMPLE PROGRAM:
DAY 1:

Dynamic Warm Up:

One Turkish Get-Up/side

Superset
> One Arm Military Press x 5 reps x 4 sets
> Single Leg Deadlift: x 5 reps/side x 4 sets

Superset:
> Renegade Row x 5 reps/side x 4 sets
> Front Squat x 5 reps x 4 sets

Calf Raise x 20
Plank x 60 seconds
Repeat 3 times

DAY 2:

Dynamic Warm Up

One Turkish Get-Up/side

Superset
>Kettlebell Floor Press x 8 reps x 4 sets
>Double Clean x 8 reps x 4 sets

Superset
>Chin-Up x 8 reps x 4 sets
>Reverse Lunge x 8 reps/side x 4 sets

Superset
>Curl x 8 x 3
>Pullover x 8 x 3
>One Arm Suitcase Carry x 50 ft/side

The sample two day program is a full body routine balanced between pushing and pulling, and between unilateral and bilateral exercises.

Cardiovascular training modalities and how to incorporate them into a program will be discussed later in this text.

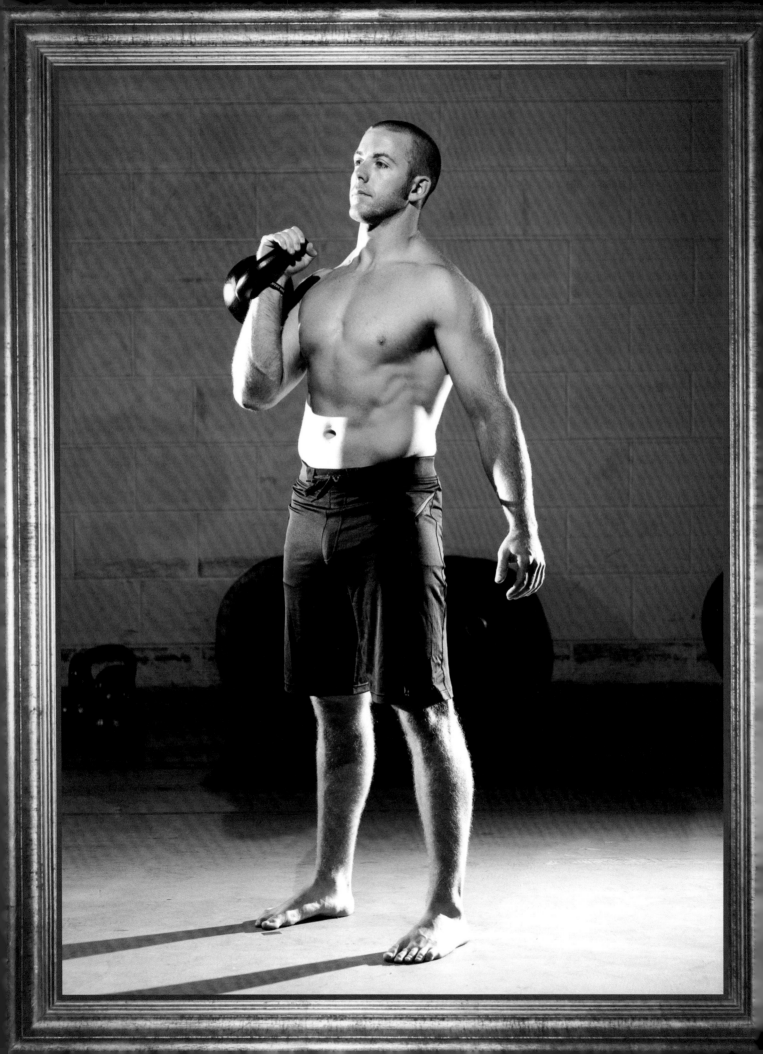

CHAPTER SIX

PROGRAM DESIGN

Most modern strength and conditioning programs are simply not well put together—they hurt people and focus on body parts rather than movement patterns. Often, the wrong movement patterns are emphasized and exacerbate common movement dysfunctions. We will take a very simple and careful approach to ensuring a balanced body through exercise.

Most people will having the same common problems:

- Frequent sitting (we can assume 4-10 hours per day)
- Stiffness in pecs and biceps (shoulders rounded forward)
- Stiffness in hip flexors and quadriceps
- Hyperactive lower back
- Poor glute and lat function

Considering the list above, it's odd that the everyday exerciser's primary focus usually includes bench press, leg press, and curls. It's no surprise that this plan will only make movement problems worse.

Instead, we can categorize movements to fit into a template that ensures a balanced training session and complete program.

Note the following:

UPPER BODY:
- Push
  — Horizontal (Push-Up or Bench Press)
  — Vertical (Press or Handstand Push-Up)

- Pull
  — Horizontal (Any Rowing Variation)
  — Vertical (Any Pull-Up Variation)

LOWER BODY:
- **Push** (Squat or Lunge)
- **Pull** (Deadlift or Swing)

All of the above can be performed bilaterally (both arms or legs) or unilaterally (one arm or leg).

The easiest way to create a balanced program is to include each of these movements in every session. Aim to perform two pulling movements for every push (two rows for every push-up) to help to balance out excessive sitting.

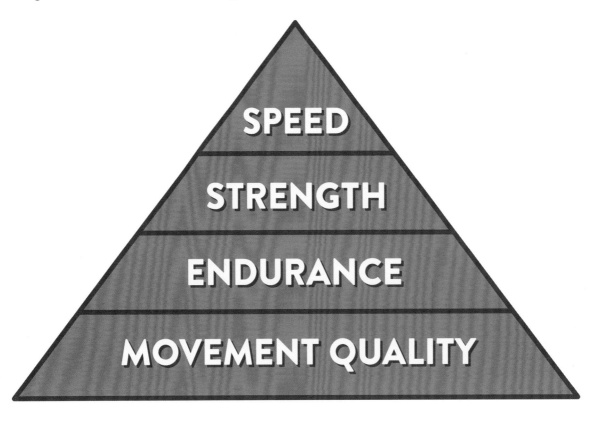

FOCUS ON MOVEMENT FIRST AND THE REST WILL EASILY FOLLOW

You need a foundation of movement quality and coordination before you can add strength and speed to it. Endurance is like a star at the top of a pyramid, once you have the other traits, it is very easy to safely acquire it—but not before the other traits.

Be realistic when planning a training program. Every day won't go as planned. Between personal life interferences and the everyday ups and downs of life, you can't expect to hit it hard every day. In fact, a person can't even be expected to train every day, let alone follow a specific plan every day. So, it makes more sense to include every movement pattern in every session instead of splitting it up. This way, if you miss a training session, you won't miss a movement pattern. In the past, it seems leg day was the easiest one to skip...

THE SIMPLE TEMPLATE:

3-5 rounds
Power
Mobility

10-20:00
Upper Push
Lower Pull
Mobility

10-20:00
Upper Pull
Lower Push
Mobility

5-10:00
Finisher/Core

This template effectively hits all the major movement patterns and athletic qualities during every session.

By pairing an upper body exercise with a lower body exercise, we can also maximize the benefit of each. Including mobility in the superset facilitates the movements or can be used as active rest. Typically you won't want to waste time with actual rest, and extra mobility work is always a good idea.

It's easier to get more practice and make faster progress by using blocks of time instead of a specific number of sets. Blocks of time allow you to take advantage of the good days by doing more reps, and take it easier with fewer reps on the days when you don't feel as strong.

This template applies not only to kettlebells but to all exercise implements including barbells or bodyweight exercises.

SAMPLE BARBELL SESSION:
Power Snatch x 3 reps x 3 sets
Mobility

Bench Press
Deadlift
Mobility

Bent Over Row
Back Squat
Mobility

Barbell Complex or Bike Intervals

SAMPLE BODYWEIGHT TRAINING SESSION:
Vertical Jump x 3 reps x 3 sets
Mobility

Handstand Push-Up
Single Leg Deadlift (unweighted)
Mobility

Pull-Up
Single Leg Squat
Mobility

Burpee Intervals

The implement isn't important—the movement is important.

GROUP TRAINING

The beauty of structuring training sessions with the template above is that it can be applied to an individual or group with no extra work. To adapt the above program for a group class, the only requirement is a clear understanding of progressions and regressions.

EXERCISE REGRESSION EXAMPLE:

One Arm Swing
Two Arm Swing
Two Arm Deadlift
Unweighted Hip Hinge (deadlift movement)

With an understanding of the progressions, it's easy to adjust the exercises to meet the different skill and strength levels within a group. This is important for keeping all group members engaged, especially those who might be at a lower strength or fitness level.

Gaining or losing weight will be primarily dictated by diet. In general, if you consume more than you expend, you will gain weight. If you consume less, you will lose weight.

MUSCLE GAIN

Books upon books have been written on the science of building muscle. Our approach is driven by some science and common sense—but we are going to keep it simple.

We gain muscle mass when our brain determines that we need more to get the job done. So, we have to cause a certain amount of stress on our muscles. This requires more total volume and heavier weights. If gaining muscle mass is the goal, the repetition range should move up from pure strength work towards the 5-8 range. The focus should be on big movements like squats, presses, and pull-ups, but if the goal is hypertrophy, include some isolation work (curls, triceps extensions). If you lift heavy and eat, you will put on muscle.

FAT LOSS

The number one reason anyone starts to exercise is fat loss. Fat loss can be tricky for some people, because fat loss really should be called lifestyle change. Finding a lifestyle that's conducive to a good physique, good health, and is also sustainable, can be a herculean task. Exercise is a big part of fat loss, but the lifestyle must be sustainable for long-term body composition change to occur.

Training for fat loss should have the following characteristics:
- **Increased heart rate**
- **Full body exercise**
- **Explosive exercise**
- **Heavy lifting**
- **Intervals of high and low intensity**

These criteria make kettlebell swings an ideal solution for fat loss. Consider swing intervals—in the Cardiovascular Training section—the perfect finisher to a strength training, fat-busting workout session.

The role of hormones in fat loss and muscle gain is often overlooked but can play a huge role in whether or not you achieve the body you want. The main factors influencing these hormones include sleep quality and quantity, nutrition (especially healthy fat intake), water intake, and stress levels. Maximizing these factors will improve the hormones that make you strong and lean.

REHABILITATION

You're not a doctor, don't try to play one on TV. However, you may be able to help yourself or someone else just by following some basic principles of movement.

First, review the mobility warm up and assessment/correction section for good starting points on movement.

Once a good foundation is established, rehabilitation mostly involves the following:

Restoring Range of Motion (ROM)
- **Soft Tissue Release**
- **Stretching**
- **Active Stretching**

Strengthening Range of Motion (ROM)

Example Problem: Tight Shoulders
Solution:
1) Work soft tissue on rotator cuff and pec with lacrosse ball
2) Thoracic mobilizations
3) Pec and lat stretches
4) Kettlebell Armbar
5) Military Press and Overhead Carry

In the example above, the range of motion is restored and then built upon. A new foundation is made before new construction.

Any painful movements should be avoided, but anything that causes an improvement in ROM should be emphasized. As mentioned previously, re-assess frequently to determine effectiveness—in the rehabilitative phase this is even more crucial.

CARDIOVASCULAR TRAINING

America has an obsession with "cardio". Spin and step classes are some of the most well attended group exercise classes. The ratio of treadmills to squat racks in a normal gym is about 40 to 1. We love "cardio."

For most people, the purpose of cardio is to have a stronger heart and lungs in the hope of longevity, increased fat burning, and overall health. Usually, we exceed the minimum effective dose with the idea that more running on a treadmill or elliptical machine is better. Often, more isn't better—it's just more.

In this book, our approach to conditioning emphasizes time management, sustainability and effectiveness. Intervals, kettlebell ballistic exercises, and bodyweight training at a moderate to high intensity will be the primary focus. Since the average exerciser has roughly less than an hour for an entire training session, conditioning will be 10 minutes or less—usually less.

INTERVAL TRAINING

Interval training simply means a period of exercise, followed by a period of active rest, repeated many times.

For example:
 30 seconds kettlebell swings
 30 seconds rest
 Repeat 5 times
 (The above is a :30/:30 kettlebell swing interval)

Intervals allow you to perform at a higher level for a longer overall duration compared to a continuous performance. In contrast, to do five minutes of continuous swings, you'd need to choose a significantly lighter kettlebell and would not be able to swing at the same intensity. The :30/:30 interval could be applied to running, and you would be able to run much faster by resting between sets. The work to rest ratio can be modified to suit not only the exercise, but the exerciser.

A stone cold beginner could do the following:
 10 seconds kettlebell swings
 50 seconds rest
 Repeat 5 times

It should be clear that the shorter the rest, the higher the potential intensity, while a longer rest will result in a lower intensity.

KETTLEBELL BALLISTICS

The kettlebell swing is the most versatile movement in this book. Performed for low reps it can be used for strength or power. High repetitions produce muscular and cardiovascular endurance. The swing should be the go-to choice for your kettlebell conditioning work. It promotes fat loss, muscular strength, and endurance in a way that few movements can match.

The kettlebell snatch, though a more risky exercise than the swing, carries many of the same benefits. If you are looking to change up the routine, include the kettlebell snatch in your regimen. The snatch is best utilized through interval training or a timed set with a goal of hitting as many reps as safely possible in a set time (3-10 minutes).

COMPLEXES

Complexes are ultimate in efficiency wrapped up in a bow. When done properly, a complex is a great way to promote strength, hypertrophy, endurance, and fat loss. A complex is a set of exercises performed without setting the implement down. Kettlebells are the ideal tool for complexes, their ergonomic design makes it easy to seamlessly transition from one movement to the next.

A great example of a kettlebell complex is the "Swing Sandwich"
   5 Double Swings
   5 Double Cleans
   5 Double Presses
   5 Double Squats
   5 Double Swings
   Rest (much needed)

During the transitions from one movement to the next, muscles are given a rest, while the heart and lungs continue to work double time. Complexes may be used for lower repetitions (1-3) to emphasize strength or higher repetitions (8+) for masochistic individuals looking for a conditioning challenge.

CHAINS

A chain is a complex where only one repetition is performed. A chain can be performed multiple times in a row without setting the implement down.

An example chain:
  1 Swing
  1 Clean
  1 Press
  1 Squat
  Repeat 5 times before switching arms and repeating on the other side.

A chain will typically result in less lactic acid or muscle fatigue than a complex due to the single repetitions. It's a fun and interesting way to change up a workout.

CALISTHENICS

The military (as early as the Spartans) has successfully used bodyweight training to promote strength and endurance. When used intelligently, the chance of injury is exceptionally low because the only load is your own bodyweight. The exercises selected are entirely dependent on the individual. What may be easy for one person might be impossible for someone else. When performing bodyweight exercises for conditioning, always choose movements that you are exceptionally proficient at—as fatigue increases, coordination and skill will begin to fail, increasing risk of injury.

Some options to consider:
- **Push-Ups**
- **Squats**
- **Lunges**
- **Pull-Ups**
- **Jumping Jacks**
- **Burpees**

SPORT SPECIFIC CONDITIONING

Don't do it.

Your job is not to invent kettlebell exercises that mimic sports movements. Use kettlebells to improve GPP (General Physical Preparedness). The best way to improve endurance for a sport is playing the actual sport. SPP—Specific Physical Preparedness—is achieved only by playing the actual sport. Understand that total body strength and coordination combined with sport practice will yield the best athlete.

HOW TO PUT IT ALL TOGETHER

The kettlebell is an exceptional tool that can help anyone achieve and surpass their fitness goals faster and more efficiently—but it is only a tool. It happens to have optimal ergonomics for specific tasks and exercises, so it should be used in these cases.

Programs should not be implement-specific, they should be movement specific. A program's exercises should be chosen based on how well they will accomplish the goal. An example would be choosing between a kettlebell press or a handstand push-up which are in the same movement category. We can categorize movements, or combine similar movements into specific categories—this transcends the implement being used. See the Program Design section for more information.

There are a few movements where a barbell or set of dumbbells is usually a better choice. Don't try to install a screw with a hammer.
- Heavy Deadlifts
- Heavy Squats
- Olympic Lifts
- Bench Press

If you already have a complete strength program but want to add kettlebell training, here's a recommendation:

Start your session with some get-ups.
Finish your session with some swings.

This is a very simple way to greatly benefit from kettlebell training. The get-ups serve as a good warm up and shoulder stability drill. The swings are excellent for conditioning as well as a form of posterior chain accessory work. Even just a small investment of time with the bells can send your strength and conditioning to new levels.

12 WEEK PROGRAM

Odd Weeks 1,3,5,7,9,11 (6-8 reps)
Even Weeks 2,4,6,8,10,12 (2-4 reps)

Each section of the training session is split into supersets and divided into time increments. Simply perform each superset of exercises for the indicated length of time before moving on to the next block of time. The interspersed mobility drills serve as active rest, and to improve flexibility with strength at the same time.

DAILY WARM UP:

Joint Circles head to toe

2 Rounds
Glute Bridge x 10
Unweighted Single-Leg Deadlift x 6/side
Lunge x 5/side
Squat x 10
Front Plank :20
Side Plank :15/side
Swing x 10
Get-Up-Arm Bar-Windmill Combo x 1/1

DAY 1:

15:00
Double Kettlebell Press
Deadlift
Side Lying Thoracic Rotation x 5/side

15:00
Row
KB Lunge
Wall Slides x 10

One Arm Swing Intervals :15 on :15 off for 5:00

DAY 2:

15:00
Push-Up or Bench Press
Single Leg Deadlift
Thoracic Rotation

15:00
Pull-Up or Chin-Up
Double KB Front Squat
Hip Flexor Stretch :15/side

One Arm Clean and Jerk Intervals
:30 left arm, rest :30
:30 right arm, rest :30
Repeat for 3-5 rounds

DAY 3:

15:00
One Arm Bottoms Up Press
Heavy Double Kettlebell Clean
Thoracic Rotation

15:00
One Arm Row
One Arm Kettlebell Front Squat
Armbar x :15/side

DAY 4:

10:00
Get-Up (1 rep per set)
Single Arm Heavy Swing

Swing Sandwich: (repeat 4 times)
Double Swing
Double Clean
Double Front Squat
Double Swing

The above program should always be done with proper technique and submaximal effort. This will ensure maximum benefits while avoiding injury.

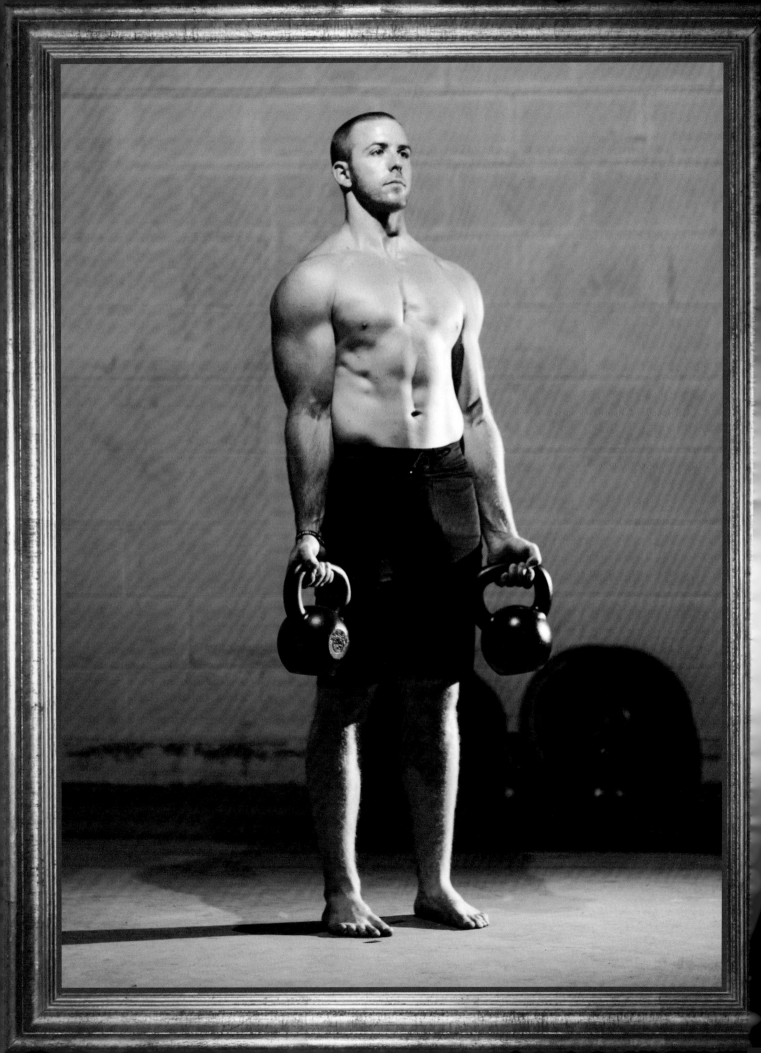

CONCLUSION

Cultivating a healthy lifestyle is a lifelong endeavor that can be made easier and more effective by using certain tools. The common denominator with any tool is you. The kettlebell is just a tool, this book is about you—what you decide to do with the kettlebell is up to you. Hopefully after reading this book, you have a much better idea of how to use it, and how to put your training together so that it fits seamlessly into your lifestyle plan.

Yours in Strength and Health,

—Max

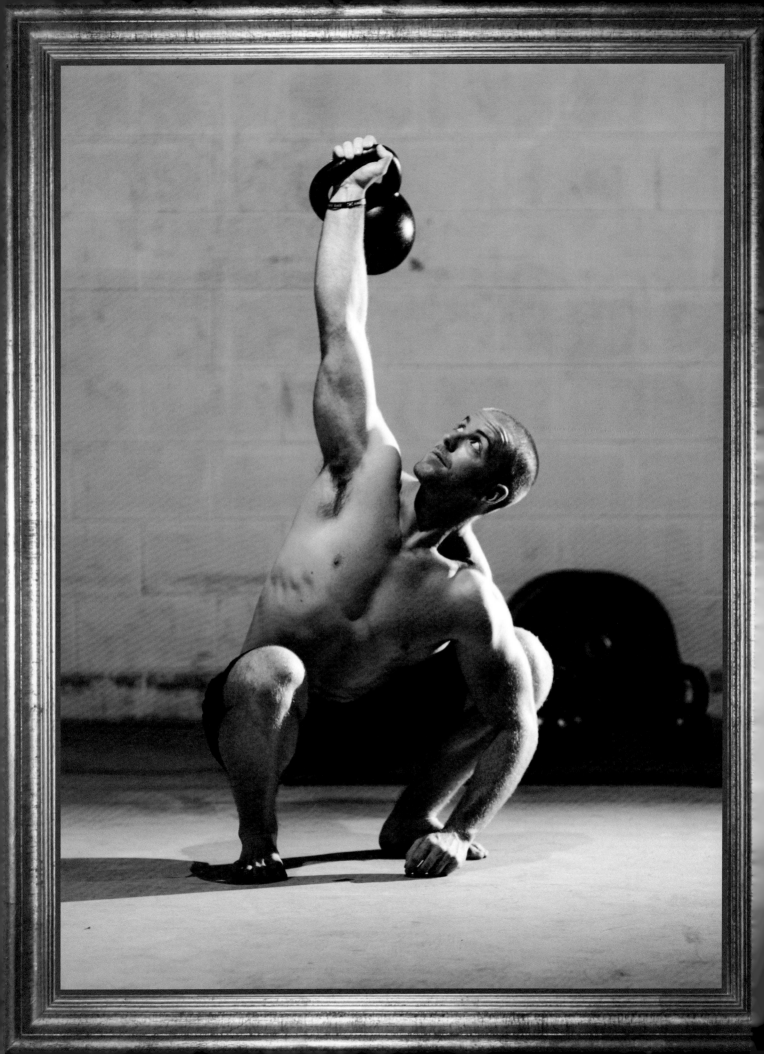

ABOUT THE AUTHOR

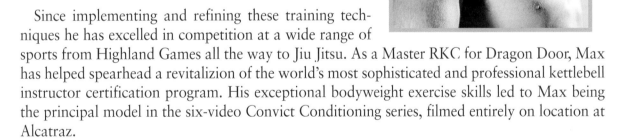

Max Shank "found" exercise at age 18, without even the ability to touch his toes or do a single pull up. Upon this discovery Max immersed himself deeply in every piece of information he could get his hands on regarding exercise, from weightlifting to gymnastics and back again. Shortly thereafter he founded Ambition Athletics, out of a desire to help make everyone better, sharing the same strategies that helped him go from "zero to hero."

Since implementing and refining these training techniques he has excelled in competition at a wide range of sports from Highland Games all the way to Jiu Jitsu. As a Master RKC for Dragon Door, Max has helped spearhead a revitalizion of the world's most sophisticated and professional kettlebell instructor certification program. His exceptional bodyweight exercise skills led to Max being the principal model in the six-video Convict Conditioning series, filmed entirely on location at Alcatraz.

Max's passion to improve his knowledge and personal skills every day has led him to be a sought after international presenter of his unique and pragmatic blend of strength, flexibility, health, and overall athleticism.

Max can be reached through his website at www.maxshank.com.

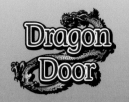
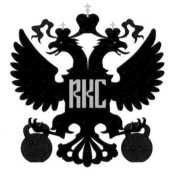
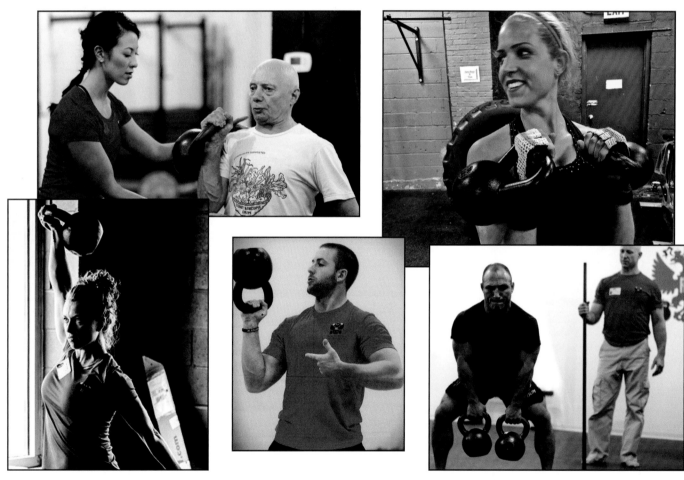

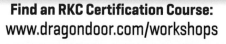

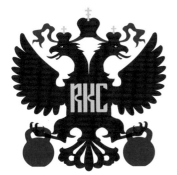

Russian Kettlebell Certification (RKC)

Dragon Door's 3-Day, Advanced Kettlebell Instructor Certification Course

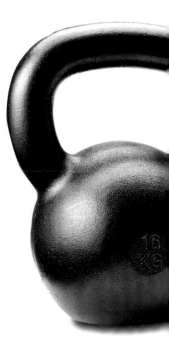

How to take your kettlebell lifting to the next level, dominate your competition, and dramatically advance your skills as a personal trainer or coach

Enhance Your Strength and Conditioning, Boost Your Income and Attract More Customers—With the RKC Advantage...

Master the essentials and dive deeper into the advanced kettlebell lifts during this comprehensive 3-day instructor course. Discover the most effective, safe, and efficient ways to use, teach and coach the core kettlebell lifts including the Swing, Get-Up, Front Squat, Military Press, Clean, and Snatch. During this hands-on course, you will be both coached and will coach others, to facilitate your learning process.

RKC's unique training protocols develop superior athleticism—by reinforcing natural movement patterns, boosting explosive power from the hips and by challenging the stabilizers during all lifts, be it ballistics or grinds. The RKC toolbox gives fitness professionals an intensive "graduate-level" arsenal of methods—guaranteed to get fast, impressive results for both their clients and for themselves.

- **Learn how** to get superior results with clients ranging from the athletic to beginners and the deconditioned
- **Enhance your skills** as a movement coach by learning how to quickly assess, correct & teach these complex movement patterns
- **Get a FREE monthly newsletter** with articles, recipes, training tips and marketing help
- **Discover how** to incorporate kettlebells into your current programming to maximize your client's results
- **Discover simple yet highly effective** cueing & troubleshooting techniques to

speed up the learning process—to get faster results for your clients

- **Learn simple techniques** for preventing and recovering from injuries
- **Get a free instructor page** on Dragon Door's website and join a community of the world's top trainers
- **Get access to the Private RKC-only Forum and network** with some of the greatest minds and coaches in the industry
- **And** as a certified RKC, you always get **20% off all Dragon Door's premium RKC kettlebells!**

Become certified as an RKC and join the world's premier community of fitness professionals!

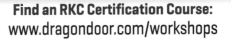

Build Your Body To Be Ripped, Rugged and Spectacular—With Dragon Door's Best-of-Class, RKC Kettlebell

The Ultimate "Handheld Gym"—Designed for A Lifetime of Hard, High-Performance Use…

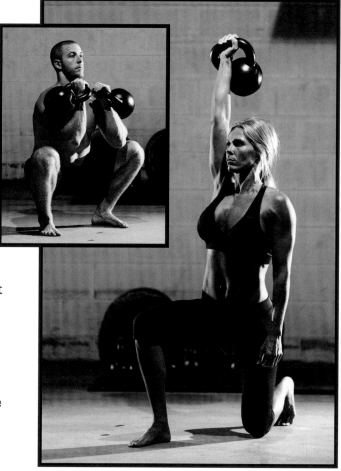

Even a man of average initial strength can immediately start using the 16kg/35lb kettlebell for two-handed swings and quickly gravitate to one-handed swings, followed by jerks, cleans and snatches. Within a few weeks you can expect to see spectacular gains in overall strength and conditioning—and for many—significant fat loss.

Dragon Door re-introduced kettlebells to the US with the uniquely designed 35lb cast iron kettlebell—and it has remained our most popular kettlebell. Why? Let Dragon Door's own satisfied customers tell the story:

Excellent Quality

"Unlike other kettlebells I have used, Dragon Door is of far superior quality. You name it, Dragon Door has got it! Where other bells lack, Dragon Door kettlebells easily meet, if not exceed, what a bell is supposed to have in quality! Great balance, nice thick handle for grip strength, and a finish that won't destroy your hands when doing kettlebell exercises."
—Barry Adamson, Frederick, MD

New Dragon Door Bells— Best Ever!

"Just received a new e-coat 16 yesterday. Perfect balance, perfect texturing, non-slip paint, and absolutely seamless."
—Daniel Fazzari, Carson City, NV

Continually Impressed

"Dragon Door never fails to impress with their quality service and products. I bought the 16kg last month and since adding it to my kettlebell 'arsenal', I am seeing huge improvement from the heavier weight. I have larger hands for a woman so the handle on the 16kg fits my hands perfectly and it feels great…This is my fifth month using kettlebells and I cannot imagine NOT using them. They have changed my life." —Tracy Ann Mangold, Combined Locks, WI

Dragon Door bells just feel better

"I purchased this 35lb bell for a friend, and as I was carrying it to him I was thinking of ways I could keep it for myself. Everything about this bell is superior to other brands. The finish is the perfect balance of smooth and rough. The handle is ample in both girth and width even for a 35 lb bell, and the shape/dimensions make overhead work so much more comfortable. There is a clear and noticeable difference between Dragon Door bells and others. Now I am looking to replace my cheap bells with Dragon Door's. On a related note, my friend is thrilled with his bell." —Raphael Sydnor, Woodberry Forest, VA

Made for Heavy-Duty Use!

"These kettlebells are definitely made for heavy-duty use! They are heftier than they appear, and the centrifugal force generated while swinging single or two-handed requires correct form. I have read numerous online reviews of different companies wh[o] manufacture kettlebells, and it I have yet to read a negative review of the kettlebells sold by Dragon Door. I have both the 35 and 44 lbs KBs, and I expect to receive a 53 lbs KB from Dragon Door by next week. And as I gain in strength and proficiency I will likely order the 72 lbs KB. If you like to be challenged physically and enjoy pushing yourself, then buy a Russian Kettlebell and start swinging!"
—Mike Davis, Newman, CA

Dragon Door Kettlebells: The Real Deal!

"The differences between Dragon Door's authentic Russian kettlebell and the inferior one which I had purchased earlier at a local big box sports store are astounding! The Dragon Door design and quality are clearly superior, and your kettlebell just 'feel[s]' right in my hand. There is absolutely no compariso[n] (and yes, I returned the substandard hunk of iron t[o] the big box store for a credit as soon as I received your kettlebell). I look forward to purchasing a heavier kettlebell from dragondoor.com as soon as [I] master the 16kg weight!"—Stephen Williams, Arlington, VA

Whatever Your Athletic Challenge, Dragon Door Has the Perfect Kettlebell Size to Meet Your Demand!

Add The Official RKC, Military-Grade Kettlebell to Your Arsenal—Durable, Resilient and Perfectly Designed to Give You Years of Explosive Gains in Strength, Endurance and Power

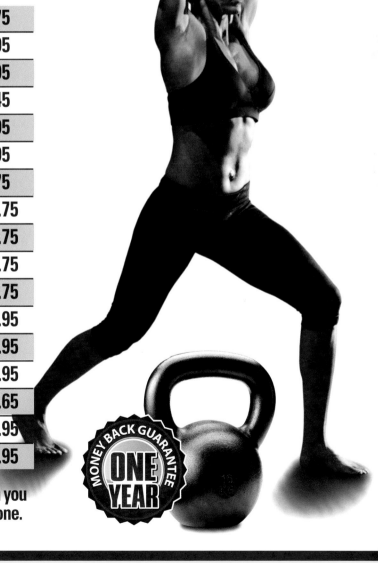

Size	Type	Item #	Price
10 lbs.	Kettlebell	#P10N	$41.75
14 lbs.	Kettlebell	#P10P	$54.95
18 lbs.	Kettlebell	#P10M	$65.95
10 kg (22 lbs.)	Kettlebell	#P10T	$71.45
12 kg (26 lbs.)	Kettlebell	#P10G	$76.95
14 kg (31 lbs.)	Kettlebell	#P10U	$87.95
16 kg (35 lbs.)	Kettlebell	#P10A	$96.75
18 kg (40 lbs.)	Kettlebell	#P10W	$102.75
20 kg (44 lbs.)	Kettlebell	#P10H	$107.75
22 kg (48 lbs.)	Kettlebell	#P10X	$112.75
24 kg (53 lbs.)	Kettlebell	#P10B	$118.75
28 kg (62 lbs.)	Kettlebell	#P10J	$142.95
32 kg (70 lbs.)	Kettlebell	#P10C	$153.95
36 kg (79 lbs.)	Kettlebell	#P10Q	$175.95
40 kg (88 lbs.)	Kettlebell	#P10F	$197.65
44 kg (97 lbs.)	Kettlebell	#P10R	$241.95
48 kg (106 lbs.)	Kettlebell	#P10L	$263.95

The appropriate shipping charge will be displayed when you order online or will be given to you when ordering by phone.

MONEY BACK GUARANTEE
ONE YEAR

CALL NOW: 1-800-899-5111 OR VISIT: www.dragondoor.com

Why the *RKC Beast Tamer* and the *RKC Iron Maiden* Define All-Around, Elite Strength—And How YOU Can Train to Master the Challenge Yourself...

In Dragon Door's RKC kettlebell instructor training system, the **Beast Tamer** and **Iron Maiden** challenges represent the ultimate athletic achievement of an elite few men and women. To earn the accolade of "Beast Tamer" men must flawlessly perform a Pistol, a Pullup and a Press—with a 108-lbs kettlebell. To earn the accolade of "Iron Maiden" women must flawlessly perform a Pistol, a Pull Up and a Press—with a 53-lbs kettlebell.

These three lifts comprise elements of strength, mobility and skill that make each different enough from the others as to make performing all three a feat worthy of great respect. The RKC ranks are filled with strong, able men and women. That only around 1% have accomplished The Beast or the Iron Maiden Challenges, speaks volumes about their difficulty.

As with any great feats of strength, success comes from a combination of dedicated training, careful programming, a clear understanding of the necessary progressions and the cultivation of particular skill-sets. Without the correct formula applied in the correct manner, the RKC Beast Tamer and RKC Iron Maiden are just not going to happen.

When **Senior RKC, Andrew Read** did a deep dive to research what exactly it took to master the Beast Tamer or Iron Maiden, he discovered some clear commonalities in the training methodologies of successful Tamers and Maidens. Success leaves clues. Andrew Read shines a masterful light on those clues, building a foolproof blueprint for the achievement of elite strength.

What works in real life to become an all-around, elite strength champion? **Andrew Read** gives you the tools, tips and techniques that can turn you from ordinary to extraordinary. Want to tap into your inner Beast or inner Iron Maiden? Bring passion, dedication and supreme determination to your training table—and you CANNOT FAIL. We look forward to welcoming down the road to the RKC Beast Tamer and RKC Iron Maiden Halls of Fame!

Discover how the magic of kettlebell exercise can keep you powerful, strong and supple—at any age...

Nothing ages us faster than the lack of regular, effective exercise. Muscles melt away, bones go brittle, posture stoops, skin sags, flab hangs—and joints creak. Pain, fear and fatigue become our constant companions.

The less you exercise, the faster you decline. However, not all exercise is created equal. Many forms of exercise may at best put you in a holding pattern, while other forms of exercise might even exacerbate your health issues.

The good news is that there is one form of exercise which can give you immeasurable health benefits, whatever your age. Regular, well-designed **kettlebell workouts** may not only reverse many symptoms of aging, but will actively contribute to building your strength and power well into your 50s, 60s, 70s and 80s.

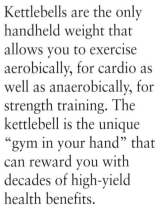

Kettlebells are the only handheld weight that allows you to exercise aerobically, for cardio as well as anaerobically, for strength training. The kettlebell is the unique "gym in your hand" that can reward you with decades of high-yield health benefits.

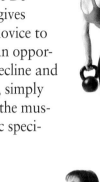

Andrea Du Cane's *The Ageless Body* presents a complete De-Aging Masterplan, that gives everyone from the raw novice to the experienced athlete an opportunity to defy physical decline and hone themselves—safely, simply and progressively—into the muscular, energetic, magnetic specimens they deserve to be.

The Ageless Body provides everything you need to start training with kettlebells, whatever your current age or condition. Bonus sections cover warm-ups, joint mobility, balance and stability—to ensure your anti-aging kettlebell program covers all the essential elements for a long, active, safe and pain-free life. Enjoy!

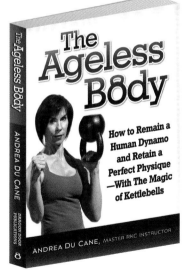

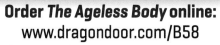

> "If you choose to reclaim your youth, look no further than *The Kettlebell Boomer.* Andrea Du Cane possesses a razor sharp mind and the kind of attention to detail that separates the high-end professionals from the also-rans. Which shall become obvious once you watch her DVD. Youth is a choice. Make it." —**Pavel Tsatsouline,** author of *Enter the Kettlebell!*

Possibly the Most Important DVD Made Since *Enter the Kettlebell!*

"Watching *The Kettlebell Boomer* reminded me of my parents and the necessity to get the transformative power of the kettlebell into the hands of the Baby Boomer Generation. This DVD will do just that.

The Kettlebell Boomer truly demonstrates that kettlebells are for EVERYBODY and no bodies need it more right now than the Boomers. This DVD is the solution to aging gracefully and it couldn't come at a better time than now. My hope is that members of the Boomer generation, with the help of my generation (Gen-X), experience what we already know - that 'when we say kettlebells, we mean strength. And when we say strength, we mean kettlebells.'"

—**GEOFF NEUPERT,** Master RKC, Durham, NC

76 million people need this DVD

"Andrea Du Cane is not a Master Instructor for nothing. She has been there from the beginning of the Kettlebell Invasion and is still leading from the front. In fact, she was my Team Leader when I got certified in 2005 and was a tough, fair and exacting instructor.

She only wanted you to do things technically correct so that you could make the best progress you could, safely. Her emphasis on technique and execution over sheer loads makes a big difference, especially when one is in the second half of their journey.

Her interest in working with the general population led her to always emphasize corrective drills, stretching, mind body connection and safety first, way before it became so popular.

Her newest DVD *The Kettlebell Boomer* is perfect for those that want a solid introduction to all the basic kb exercises as well as progressions and techniques that let them go slowly into this brave and perhaps scary new world of the kettlebell.

Given that there are 76 million people in this age range this is a product that needed to be made.

One of the charges we ask of ourselves when certifying potential RKCs is whether we would feel safe having them train our mothers. With this DVD

any instructor will have even more tools to safely bring deconditioned, older people into the kettlebell community with confidence."

—**MARK REIFKIND,** Master Instructor RKC, San Jose, CA

Excellent DVD

"*The Kettlebell Boomer* by Andrea Du Cane is full of excellent progressions, variations and techniques targeted at the 'senior' population.

Trainers will want this product so they can effectively integrate the Kettlebell into the routines of their 'senior' clients and Seniors will want this product to enhance their own Kettlebell practice or to enter into Kettlebell training. With 4 experience levels, the 'self screen' and the variations and progressions provided, this DVD can open the world of KB training to the older clientele."

—**BRETT JONES,** Master RKC, CSCS, CK-FMS, Pittsburgh, PA

What You Should Know About Andrea Du Cane and The Kettlebell Boomer

"Have you ever wondered how to overcome your physical limitations (or your clients') to optimize your performance and get real results from your kettlebell workouts?

When I owned my gym, 90% of my clients were boomers who came to me with some sort of pre-existing injury or impingement that limited the progress we could make together. Of course as an RKC, I had some tools in my toolbox to help them make breakthroughs, but I didn't have *The Kettlebell Boomer.* I remember both of us walking out of some training sessions frustrated that we didn't make the progress we intended to make. Has this ever been you?

If the answer is yes, you have to watch *The Kettlebell Boomer* with Master RKC, Andrea Du Cane. Du Cane's DVD is one of the most important kettlebell DVDs available for both trainers and kettlebell enthusiasts—here is why:

Students in the DVD are varied in their limitations and you will find either yourself or your client in this DVD.

Du Cane teaches you with sound methods how to work within and even overcome limitations.

You will learn how to reverse the effects of aging in a easy to understand format—Du Cane is professional and engaging.

Complete and thorough instruction on how to adapt certain exercises to specific limitations.

Du Cane demonstrates how to shatter plateaus, boost performance and maximize results!

Did you know boomers are estimated to be 80 million strong by 2020? As a trainer you must know how to train this group of people and as a boomer you should know that you don't need to be limited in your kettlebell training.

What was the experience you had recently that left you feeling frustrated after a training session? I am willing to bet that after you watch *The Kettlebell Boomer* you will no longer feel like you (or your client) just didn't do enough or that you (or your client) just can't perform certain kettlebell exercises. Get *The Kettlebell Boomer* now!"

—**SARAH LURIE,** Author of Kettlebells For Dummies, Montecito, CA

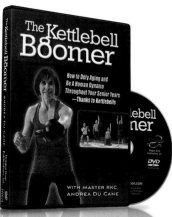

1 Beginner

2 Mid-Level

3 Advanced

The Kettlebell Boomer
How to Defy Aging and Be a Human Dynamo Throughout Your Senior Years— Thanks to Kettlebells
With Master RKC, Andrea Du Cane
#DV074 $39.95
Running time: 2 hours 50 minutes

"Stay Strong, Young, Toned and Vibrant With Andrea Du Cane's High-Powered, Super-High-Energy Kettlebell Cardio and Strength Workouts"

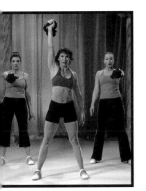

The ancient Greek Goddesses were famous for their vigorous and vibrant strength, their power, their grace and their physical elegance.

Now you have a realistic chance to make even a Greek Goddess green with envy as you match—if not surpass—them for athletic grace and high performance!

In this superbly produced, interactive, menu-based DVD, **Senior Russian Kettlebell Instructor,** *Andrea Du Cane* challenges and inspires you to seize that ideal of elegant strength and make it your own.

Andrea's powerful array of authentic kettlebell workouts, plus cool downs and stretches, are guaranteed to reward you with greater energy, greater well being, greater strength and a superb figure. Fit for the Goddess you know you are!

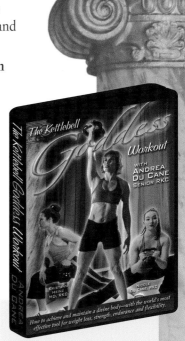

Choose from a wide variety of **Upper Body, Lower Body, Abs** and **Cardio** workouts, then mix and match to create your own customized training program for godly perfection. Your results will be strictly divine…

Or simply follow along with one of the six **Goddess Workouts** for a complete, carefully targeted session designed to carve away the fat and sculpt lean, toned muscles—ready and willing to take on the world and win it all. Just like Athena… Just like Nike…

Once the hard-kept secret of elite Russian athletes, special forces and 'manly' men, the kettlebell is now becoming the preferred tool for women who are tired of being merely human and tired of mediocre results—and who demand fast fat loss, high energy and exceptional physical performance, now! Let Andrea show you the way…

- **Receive** inspiring, first-class personal instruction from one of the nation's top female kettlebell athletes.

- **Renew** yourself with a constant variety of targeted, high-yield workouts that meet your changing needs.

- **Redefine** your body and exceed your mortal limits, with the divine challenge of Andrea's patented *Goddess Workouts*.

Includes a **Special Bonus Section** of additional drills to add further variety and power to your workouts.

Contents include a PDF on **How to Get the Most Out of Your** *Kettlebell Goddess Workout* DVD—plus special programming tips.

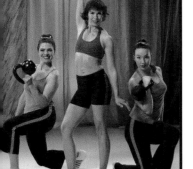

The Kettlebell Goddess Workout

Andrea Du Cane, Master RKC with Kristann Heinz, MD, RKC and Nicole Du Cane, RKC

Running time:
2 Hours and 25 minutes
DVD #DV040 $29.95

1 Beginner
2 Mid-Level
3 Advanced

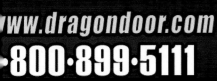

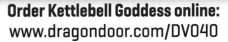

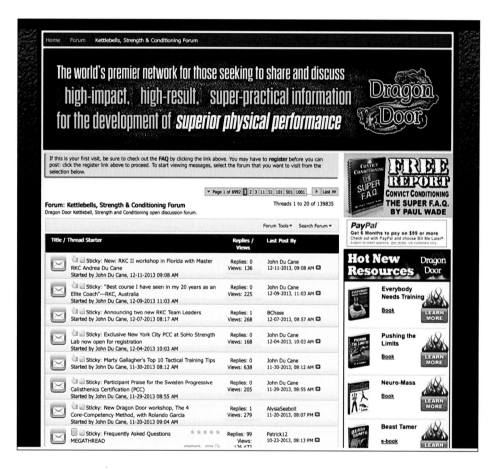

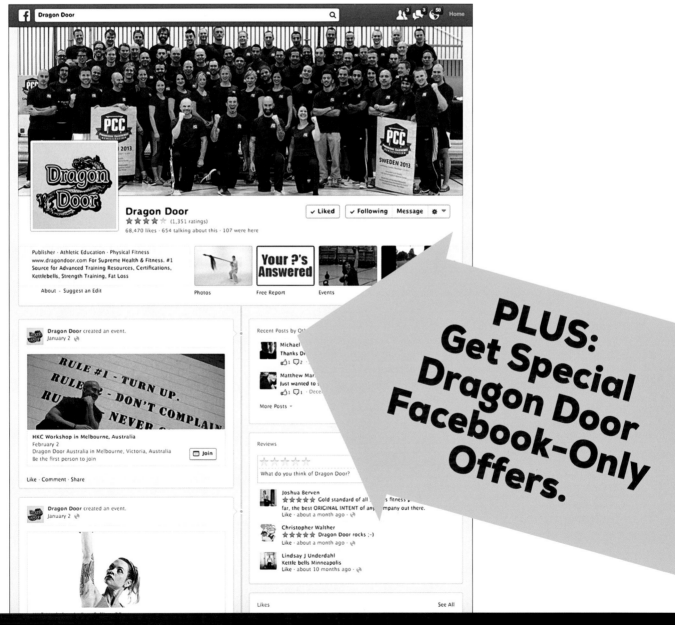

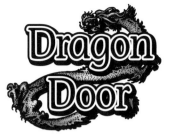

1·800·899·5111
24 HOURS A DAY • FAX YOUR ORDER (866) 280-7619
O R D E R I N G   I N F O R M A T I O N

Telephone Orders For faster service you may place your orders by calling Toll Free 24 hours a day, 7 days a week, 365 days per year. When you call, please have your credit card ready.

Customer Service Questions? Please call us between 9:00am– 11:00pm EST

Monday to Friday at 1-800-899-5111. Local and foreign customers call 513-346-4160 for orders and customer service

100% One-Year Risk-Free Guarantee. If you are not completely satisfied with any product—we'll be happy to give you a prompt exchange, credit, or refund, as

you wish. Simply return your purchase to us, and please let us know why you were dissatisfied—it will help us to provide better products and services in the future. *Shipping and handling fees are non-refundable.*

Complete and mail with full payment to: Dragon Door Publications, 5 County Road B East, Suite 3, Little Canada, MN 55117

Please print clearly

Sold To: A

Name_____

Street_____

City_____

State_____ Zip _____

Day phone*_____
* *Important for clarifying questions on orders*

Please print clearly

SHIP TO: *(Street address for delivery)*   B

Name_____

Street_____

City_____

State_____ Zip _____

Email_____

Warning to foreign customers:
The Customs in your country may or may not tax or otherwise charge you an additional fee for goods you receive. Dragon Door Publications is charging you only for U.S. handling and international shipping. Dragon Door Publications is in no way responsible for any additional fees levied by Customs, the carrier or any other entity.

ITEM #	QTY.	ITEM DESCRIPTION	ITEM PRICE	A OR B	TOTAL

HANDLING AND SHIPPING CHARGES • NO COD'S
Total Amount of Order Add (Excludes kettlebells and kettlebell kits):

$00.00 to 29.99	Add $6.00	$100.00 to 129.99	Add $14.00
$30.00 to 49.99	Add $7.00	$130.00 to 169.99	Add $16.00
$50.00 to 69.99	Add $8.00	$170.00 to 199.99	Add $18.00
$70.00 to 99.99	Add $11.00	$200.00 to 299.99	Add $20.00
		$300.00 and up	Add $24.00

Canada and Mexico add $6.00 to US charges. All other countries, flat rate, double US Charges. See Kettlebell section for Kettlebell Shipping and handling charges.

Total of Goods	
Shipping Charges	
Rush Charges	
Kettlebell Shipping Charges	
OH residents add 6.5% sales tax	
MN residents add 6.5% sales tax	
TOTAL ENCLOSED	

METHOD OF PAYMENT ☐ CHECK ☐ M.O. ☐ MASTERCARD ☐ VISA ☐ DISCOVER ☐ AMEX

Account No. *(Please indicate all the numbers on your credit card)*   EXPIRATION DATE

☐☐☐☐ ☐☐☐☐ ☐☐☐☐ ☐☐☐☐   ☐☐/☐☐

Day Phone: (___)_____

Signature: _____ **Date:** _____

NOTE: *We ship best method available for your delivery address. Foreign orders are sent by air. Credit card or International M.O. only. For* **RUSH** *processing of your order, add an additional $10.00 per address. Available on money order & charge card orders only.*

Errors and omissions excepted. Prices subject to change without notice.

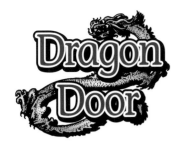

1·800·899·5111
24 HOURS A DAY • FAX YOUR ORDER (866) 280-7619
O R D E R I N G   I N F O R M A T I O N

Telephone Orders For faster service you may place your orders by calling Toll Free 24 hours a day, 7 days a week, 365 days per year. When you call, please have your credit card ready.

Customer Service Questions? Please call us between 9:00am– 11:00pm EST

Monday to Friday at 1-800-899-5111. Local and foreign customers call 513-346-4160 for orders and customer service

100% One-Year Risk-Free Guarantee. If you are not completely satisfied with any product—we'll be happy to give you a prompt exchange, credit, or refund, as

you wish. Simply return your purchase to us, and please let us know why you were dissatisfied—it will help us to provide better products and services in the future. *Shipping and handling fees are non-refundable.*

Complete and mail with full payment to: Dragon Door Publications, 5 County Road B East, Suite 3, Little Canada, MN 55117

Please print clearly

Sold To: A

Name_____

Street_____

City_____

State _____ Zip _____

Day phone*_____
* Important for clarifying questions on orders

Please print clearly

SHIP TO: *(Street address for delivery)*   B

Name_____

Street_____

City_____

State _____ Zip _____

Email_____

Warning to foreign customers:
The Customs in your country may or may not tax or otherwise charge you an additional fee for goods you receive. Dragon Door Publications is charging you only for U.S. handling and international shipping. Dragon Door Publications is in no way responsible for any additional fees levied by Customs, the carrier or any other entity.

ITEM #	QTY.	ITEM DESCRIPTION	ITEM PRICE	A OR B	TOTAL

HANDLING AND SHIPPING CHARGES • NO COD'S
Total Amount of Order Add (Excludes kettlebells and kettlebell kits):

$00.00 to 29.99	Add $6.00	$100.00 to 129.99	Add $14.00
$30.00 to 49.99	Add $7.00	$130.00 to 169.99	Add $16.00
$50.00 to 69.99	Add $8.00	$170.00 to 199.99	Add $18.00
$70.00 to 99.99	Add $11.00	$200.00 to 299.99	Add $20.00
		$300.00 and up	Add $24.00

Canada and Mexico add $6.00 to US charges. All other countries, flat rate, double US Charges. See Kettlebell section for Kettlebell Shipping and handling charges.

Total of Goods	
Shipping Charges	
Rush Charges	
Kettlebell Shipping Charges	
OH residents add 6.5% sales tax	
MN residents add 6.5% sales tax	
TOTAL ENCLOSED	

METHOD OF PAYMENT ❑ CHECK ❑ M.O. ❑ MASTERCARD ❑ VISA ❑ DISCOVER ❑ AMEX

Account No. *(Please indicate all the numbers on your credit card)*   EXPIRATION DATE

☐☐☐☐ ☐☐☐☐ ☐☐☐☐ ☐☐☐☐   ☐☐/☐☐

Day Phone: (___)_____
Signature: _____ **Date:** _____

NOTE: *We ship best method available for your delivery address. Foreign orders are sent by air. Credit card or International M.O. only. For **RUSH** processing of your order, add an additional $10.00 per address. Available on money order & charge card orders only.*

Errors and omissions excepted. Prices subject to change without notice.

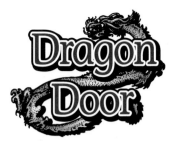

1·800·899·5111
24 HOURS A DAY • FAX YOUR ORDER (866) 280-7619
ORDERING INFORMATION

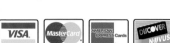

Telephone Orders For faster service you may place your orders by calling Toll Free 24 hours a day, 7 days a week, 365 days per year. When you call, please have your credit card ready.

Customer Service Questions? Please call us between 9:00am– 11:00pm EST

Monday to Friday at 1-800-899-5111. Local and foreign customers call 513-346-4160 for orders and customer service

100% One-Year Risk-Free Guarantee. If you are not completely satisfied with any product—we'll be happy to give you a prompt exchange, credit, or refund, as

you wish. Simply return your purchase to us, and please let us know why you were dissatisfied—it will help us to provide better products and services in the future. *Shipping and handling fees are non-refundable.*

Complete and mail with full payment to: Dragon Door Publications, 5 County Road B East, Suite 3, Little Canada, MN 55117

Please print clearly

Sold To: **A**

Name_____

Street_____

City_____

State _____ Zip _____

Day phone*_____
* *Important for clarifying questions on orders*

Please print clearly

SHIP TO: *(Street address for delivery)*   **B**

Name_____

Street_____

City_____

State _____ Zip _____

Email_____

Warning to foreign customers:
The Customs in your country may or may not tax or otherwise charge you an additional fee for goods you receive. Dragon Door Publications is charging you only for U.S. handling and international shipping. Dragon Door Publications is in no way responsible for any additional fees levied by Customs, the carrier or any other entity.

ITEM #	QTY.	ITEM DESCRIPTION	ITEM PRICE	A OR B	TOTAL

HANDLING AND SHIPPING CHARGES • NO COD'S
Total Amount of Order Add (Excludes kettlebells and kettlebell kits):

$00.00 to 29.99	Add $6.00	$100.00 to 129.99	Add $14.00
$30.00 to 49.99	Add $7.00	$130.00 to 169.99	Add $16.00
$50.00 to 69.99	Add $8.00	$170.00 to 199.99	Add $18.00
$70.00 to 99.99	Add $11.00	$200.00 to 299.99	Add $20.00
		$300.00 and up	Add $24.00

Canada and Mexico add $6.00 to US charges. All other countries, flat rate, double US Charges. See Kettlebell section for Kettlebell Shipping and handling charges.

Total of Goods	
Shipping Charges	
Rush Charges	
Kettlebell Shipping Charges	
OH residents add 6.5% sales tax	
MN residents add 6.5% sales tax	
TOTAL ENCLOSED	

METHOD OF PAYMENT ❑ CHECK ❑ M.O. ❑ MASTERCARD ❑ VISA ❑ DISCOVER ❑ AMEX

Account No. *(Please indicate all the numbers on your credit card)*   EXPIRATION DATE

⬜⬜⬜⬜ ⬜⬜⬜⬜ ⬜⬜⬜⬜ ⬜⬜⬜⬜   ⬜⬜/⬜⬜

Day Phone: (____)_____

Signature: _____   **Date:** _____

NOTE: *We ship best method available for your delivery address. Foreign orders are sent by air. Credit card or International M.O. only. For* **RUSH** *processing of your order, add an additional $10.00 per address. Available on money order & charge card orders only.*

Errors and omissions excepted. Prices subject to change without notice.